PHYSICIAN OR MAGICIAN?

THE MYTHS AND REALITIES OF PATIENT CARE

B. F. Fuller, M.D.
Clinical Professor of Medicine
University of Minnesota Medical School

Frank Fuller

With a foreword by
Donald M. Fraser
U.S. House of Representatives

HEMISPHERE PUBLISHING CORPORATION
Washington London

McGRAW-HILL BOOK COMPANY
New York St. Louis San Francisco Auckland Bogotá
Düsseldorf Johannesburg London Madrid Mexico
Montreal New Delhi Panama Paris São Paulo
Singapore Sydney Tokyo Toronto

PHYSICIAN OR MAGICIAN? The Myths and Realities of Patient Care

1 2 3 4 5 6 7 8 9 0 MUMU 7 8 3 2 1 0 9 8

This book was set in Century Medium by Hemisphere Publishing Corporation. The editors were F. P. Begell, Rolfe W. Larson, and Mary Dorfman; the designer was Lilia N. Guerrero; the production supervisor was Rebekah McKinney.
The Murray Printing Company was printer and binder.

Library of Congress Cataloging in Publication Data

Fuller, Benjamin F., date.
Physician or magician?

Includes index.
1. Physician and patient. 2. Physicians.
I. Fuller, Frank, date, joint author.
II. Title. [DNLM: 1. Physician—Patient relations.
2. Patient care planning. 3. Primary health care.
W62 F965p]
R727.3.F84 610.69'6 78-3625
ISBN 0-07-022617-2

Contents

Foreword

Dr. Fuller's subject is a timely one. Medical advances, he observes, have complicated the physician's function to treat the whole person. The very technological advances that have made medical care more effective have, ironically, caused the major problems that beset medical care today—high costs, inefficiency, inaccessibility, and imbalance. While technology has increasingly dominated medical care, the relationship between doctor and patient has become more remote. Excessive use of technology, moreover, has led the patient to expect magical medical cures.

Dr. Fuller offers alternative approaches that may be used to reverse the trend away from primary, total care practice. To remedy the failure of the medical profession to treat the whole person, he recommends sweeping changes in the education of physicians and emphasizes the need to clarify and redefine the physician's role and function. He calls for the training and development of physicians in two distinct categories—conceptually oriented, or primary care, physicians and technologically oriented physicians.

The primary care physician envisioned by Dr. Fuller would be responsible for the total, long-term continuing care of the patient. The main commodity of the primary physician, he stresses, should be decisions—about the kind and number of diagnostic studies necessary, whether specialists are needed, the nature of treatment, and the extent of treatment. Technologically oriented physicians would be limited to consultations, specialized treatment, and surgery. The primary physician, in Dr. Fuller's view, must become a manager, a data gatherer, an interpreter and evaluator, a decision maker, a probability expert, and a therapist.

This book is an appeal for an informed public that will work through the political establishment to help make decisions about the direction of patient care. At a time when the federal government is exploring new approaches in the way we deliver and pay for health care services, Dr. Fuller has focused on the important and neglected question of providing more humane and more patient-oriented health care. His ideas merit special attention and discussion.

Donald M. Fraser
U.S. House of Representatives
Minnesota, Fifth District

Preface

This book is the product of thirty-five years of observation of the medical–social–political scene. During those thirty-five years, my vantage point has changed from medical student to medical fellow to medical officer in the Armed Forces to private practitioner to medical educator and back again to private practitioner. Sometimes, during those years, I had the feeling that I was even acting as a medical politician.

The practice of medicine has changed a great deal during my lifetime, in many ways for the better. However, not all the changes have been for the better. The advances in medical knowledge since World War II have increased the effectiveness of patient care but have, at the same time, caused many of today's problems to develop. It is difficult to pick up a newspaper or magazine today without reading about them.

As a result, solutions are being offered from a variety of sources. Some of the suggested solutions are political, some are economic, and some are attempts to manipulate the basic structure of the health care system.

As with any crisis, there is a variety of opinion about what should be done. Ultimately, choices will have to be made from among these opinions. It is probable that many of the choices will be made by the elected representatives of the public as they interpret the desires of their constituents.

During my years in medical practice, I learned many

things from my patients. One of these was that most patients, if they are provided with the necessary information, are able to make the most difficult decisions. Most important, they are able to do this well. I have rarely been disappointed in this impressive capacity of patients. However, it is critical that they be provided with accurate information.

That is why I wrote this book. As I look at suggested solutions to many of today's health care problems, I find some of them appealing and some frightening. Since I believe that the public will have the ultimate responsibility for choosing among them, I have attempted in this book to provide what I perceive to be important and necessary information for making such choices. My concern is preservation of the quality of care. This book defines what I believe to be essential ingredients of quality.

Acknowledging help received is virtually an impossible task because one's positions are determined by one's total life experience. The inevitable result is that the thoughts presented in this book are the product of all the interactions of my lifetime with family, friends, teachers, patients, students, and colleagues.

In addition to the above, I received valuable advice from a number of colleagues and friends who reviewed this manuscript for me during its formative stages. These people included Wallace D. Armstrong, Walter W. Benjamin, Kjeld O. Husebye, Sherod L. Miller, John S. Millis, Thomas J. Rose, Vernon E. Weckwerth, and Milton D. Zeddies.

I am particularly indebted to John S. Millis, not only for reviewing the manuscript, but also for being a major influence in my decision to author this book.

First person singular pronouns are used throughout this book. All such references are to me, Dr. B. F. Fuller. The content of this book is derived from my experience as a private practitioner and medical educator. Frank Fuller organized the material and wrote the book.

B. F. Fuller

Introduction 1

Neither do men put new wine into old wineskins: else the skins burst, and the wine is spilled and the skins perish: but they put new wine into fresh wineskins and both are preserved.

Matt. 9:17

The parable cited above was used by Arnold Toynbee in a discussion of "social enormities" in *A Study of History*.[1] A social enormity, he wrote, is an institution that has become an anachronism because it is expected to perform in a manner for which it was never intended. He cited the parable to warn that an anachronistic institution is unable to respond to forces and pressures that were never envisioned while the institution was developing. So, as society changes, old institutions must adapt to the new times or else they will shatter and be pushed aside.

We are approaching this point in the medical profession in the United States. As more and more methods of changing the institution are suggested, it becomes more and more like another of Toynbee's examples, an old steam engine that is expected to perform in ways for which it was never intended. A new head of steam could destroy the engine. The medical profession needs change, but people must be concerned that the most desirable parts of the

[1] Arnold J. Toynbee, *A Study of History*, Oxford University Press, New York, 1947.

system may be destroyed along with less desirable parts unless the changes are carefully selected.

The quality of patient care should be the focus of all discussions because if the entire institution were destroyed, the high technical quality of patient care in the United States—and it is the best in the world—could be lost forever. This could happen within one generation. Yet it is understandable why discussions do not center on this issue. Most people outside the profession do not understand the function of physicians. In fact, even within the profession, relatively few people have been trying to define the physician's function.

Both outside and inside the profession, most of the suggested changes have centered around the inflated cost of health care. Price ceilings have been set, national insurance programs have been suggested, and physician substitutes are being trained and used. But none of these suggestions deals at all with the quality of patient care—how to maintain it at its present level or improve it while containing cost. Physician substitutes, for example, while well-trained in a specific field, do not have the same expertise that physicians *should* have and that most physicians *do* have. A well-educated physician is better prepared to evaluate the diverse and complex questions raised by patients on a day-to-day basis.

If the changes come from within the medical profession, and that implies a revolutionary change in its hierarchical structure including redefinition of responsibility and authority in patient care, the profession will take a major step toward adapting to the present needs of society. This will require a change of emphasis in the education of physicians, which, one hopes, will lead to change in the daily practice of physicians.

Many in the health care system disagree over what changes are necessary. In fact, these disagreements have gone on for quite a few years. It is time that the public is apprised of some of these issues. Then, let us all hope that an informed public will take positions that ensure that the present high quality of patient care will be preserved and even improved.

Several years ago, I was asked to see an elderly woman whose immediate medical problem was due to a circulatory disease. The circulation to both legs was severely impaired, and gangrenous changes had occurred in the skin of both feet. In addition, she had been confined to a wheelchair for several years with severe arthritis.

I was asked for an opinion concerning whether surgery might help reestablish the flow of blood to her legs and feet. After examining the patient and reviewing the data on her chart, I came to the following conclusions:

1. The circulatory disease had advanced to the point where the likelihood of surgically restoring circulation was quite small;
2. The patient's general condition would probably confine her to a wheelchair for the rest of her life, even if circulation could be restored to her legs;
3. Attempting to surgically restore circulation to a severely diseased extremity of this type frequently results in performing multiple surgical procedures sequentially; and
4. The possible benefit to this patient (even if the surgery were successful) was small, and the potential risk of surgical complications and/or prolonged hospitalization was great.

Therefore, I recommended amputation of both legs, one above the knee and one below the knee.

Several days later, I was asked to see the patient again.

An arteriogram (an X-ray of an artery, which demonstrates whether and to what extent the artery is obstructed) confirmed my opinion that the circulatory disease in one leg was uncorrectable. It also showed that the arterial disease in the other leg was advanced and probably uncorrectable. It did, however, introduce slight doubt by suggesting that there was a remote possibility that reconstructive surgery might improve the circulation in one leg by a small amount.

On the basis of this X-ray, it was decided to amputate one leg and to attempt to repair the circulatory problem in the other leg. This decision was not made lightly. It was preceded by a conference that lasted an hour and a half and that was attended by all the physicians involved in the care of this patient. Two positions were taken at the conference. One was that both legs should be amputated because the chance of restoring circulation to either leg continued to be so small that the risk of attempting surgical repair would not be justified. The prevailing view was that one leg should be amputated, but that surgery should be performed to attempt to restore circulation to the other leg before amputation of that leg was considered.

The patient was in the hospital for four and one-half months, during which she had five surgical procedures as well as postoperative pneumonia, thrombophlebitis, and pulmonary embolism. The final result was that both legs had been amputated, one above the knee and one below the knee. She was then discharged to nursing home care. The hospital bill (not including the physicians' fees) exceeded $18,000. The patient was demoralized during the hospitalization.

It should be pointed out that all of the physicians involved in the decisions concerning this patient were extremely knowledgeable about and experienced in the diagnosis and treatment of this type of circulatory disease.

They were all held in high esteem by their colleagues, and most of their patients were referred to them by other physicians. The failure in decision making was not caused by lack of understanding of either the extent or the mechanism of the disease.

What did go wrong then? That is what this book is about.

The Problem 2

There were other tests, some of which seemed to me to be more an assertion of the clinical capability of the hospital than of concern for the well-being of the patient.

Norman Cousins, *Saturday Review*

The problems of the patient in Chapter 1, as serious as they were, did not justify the length and cost of her hospitalization, nor did they justify the complex and extensive forms of treatment used. This is easy to say when provided with the wisdom of hindsight. It must be remembered, however, that from the outset some of the physicians involved in her care recommended a different course of action, which, if it had been followed, would probably have avoided the many complications that occurred.

Does this mean that some of these physicians were competent and that the others were incompetent? Not at all. What it means is that this particular patient presented all of the physicians involved in her care with an extremely difficult dilemma and that, because of their educational and experiential backgrounds, some kinds of physicians are better equipped to handle such dilemmas than are other kinds of physicians. Decision making is the major challenge in patient care today. If the physician most directly responsible for the care of this patient had been given authority commensurate with the professional responsibility, the subsequent treatment would certainly have been different and would probably have been better for the patient. When there is disagreement among physicians, the alternative processes for resolving the resulting problems are limited. Of the various alternatives, one of the least satisfactory, from the point of view of the patient, is resolution by consensus.

Most of the dilemmas that occur in day-to-day medical practice are less dramatic and less difficult of resolution. Finding answers to simpler dilemmas, however, is in some ways even more important than resolving more complex ones. This is because they occur so frequently.

The inability of some physicians to satisfactorily deal with dilemmas may be one of the reasons for public hostility toward the medical profession. The public outcry is not entirely without cause. Doctors, after all, seem remote; in the office they may seem distant, and outside the office they have few social contacts with their patients. They tend to respond to criticism with defensiveness. Some doctors condescend to patients, not giving them credit for the ability to understand scientific explanations. People may wait an hour and then see a doctor for only five minutes, and in five minutes can a doctor answer, let alone define, the questions a patient asks?

To the physician's credit, however, the irritations a patient faces when visiting a doctor's office or a crowded clinic may be minor compared to the services the physician provides. The miracle of modern medicine is that many aches, pains, disabilities, and fears vanish shortly after a visit to a doctor. But if something goes wrong the successes are forgotten, and the minor complaints combine in a chorus demanding that something be done.

In a sense, medicine has a dual personality. On the one hand, there are the technological advances that have eradicated or controlled so many death-causing illnesses. Physicians are well-trained in the uses of technology, and no one complains when the cost is reasonable and the treatment is effective. This side of medicine is the most publicized; it hits the headlines and is dramatized on television. On the other hand, there are physicians who consider medicine to be treatment of the total person. They also use technology but attempt to do so judiciously and sparingly, not simply because it is available. They know that, in many instances, its use should be limited or avoided.

Still, there is a tendency among physicians to do whatever they can, whether it is trying to save a patient's leg at an exorbitant financial and emotional cost, or ordering extra laboratory tests for a patient who has a minor ailment. One physician may immediately utilize the available technology, another may ponder the issue before deciding, and a third may reject it. Whatever the case, the end result is too often an overuse of resources and an increase in cost.

Physicians do this partly because of the complexity of their work. Symptoms vary, descriptions of symptoms vary, causes of symptoms vary, and responses to medication vary. A physician has the option of treating each patient as a unique individual and using judgment to determine what the patient's problem is. This involves probing deeply into the patient's history. Or, the physician can partially control the data that are collected and reduce the number of possibilities without recognizing the uniqueness of the patient's problem. This will frequently result in making the patient's symptoms fit the diagnosis. The problem will be reduced to a more manageable level—such as an organ system—and the physician will then attempt to treat that problem. The total patient may be forgotten when this happens.

Throughout history, physicians have been expected to treat the total patient, not just a small portion of the patient. However, the medical advances of recent decades have complicated the physician's function. Reducing problems to a simpler level was found to be one effective way to handle a complicated situation, but physicians must also be able to resolve a complex situation. The human body is, after all, unbelievably complex, as is shown by the variety of combinations of symptoms that patients bring to a physician's office.

There are three things a physician should consider before making any decisions concerning a patient. All of them should be considered because of the risks of some of the new medical advances. The first is the risk to the life of the patient entailed by either doing something or not doing it (diagnostic testing or treatment). The second is the suffering that may result. The third is the dollar cost. The total cost to the patient should, in fact, be defined by these three variables. If they were always considered carefully, we would be able to measure the effectiveness of physicians more accurately.

Even though total cost is influenced by the physician's ability to make decisions in a dynamic situation, physicians do not always have to consider cost or abide by its implications. In other words, they do not always have to be accountable for their decisions. Buying medical care is not like buying other products; what is bought cannot be compared with what other consumers have bought. Because of this, the patient is at a disadvantage; everything the physician does that is important—diagnosis and determination of treatment—is frequently beyond the patient's understanding.

Patients' expectations also influence physician behavior. Not only do patients want to be cured or comforted, but also many expect the physician to do something visible in order to achieve this end result. Patients are aware of the medical arsenal and often want to be treated with some part of it regardless of whether their problem calls for such treatment. For example, a physician may discern that a patient wants a cast on a small chip fracture and, even though it is unnecessary, may place a cast on the extremity. Or, a physician may prescribe drugs that are either unnecessary or inert just because the patient has subtly suggested their importance. The risks are low in many of these situations, and so are the dollar costs to individual patients (although the aggregate cost is very high). Yet the fact that they occur betrays a state of mind: the physician is willing to do things that are unnecessary and useless in certain situations. One can extrapolate from this to more drastic measures, ones that increase the total cost to each patient as well as to society at large.

The results are well publicized. Costs have increased; physicians and patients seem to have unrealistic expectations, since ailments are reduced to simpler levels of organ systems and cells; and patients frequently feel dehumanized.

Let's look at cost first. This has become a major concern to the public. Health care expenditures were $3.6 billion in 1929, $12 billion in 1950, and $104 billion in 1974. These amounts represented 3.6, 4.6, and 7.7 percent of the gross national product in those years.[1] A total of $139 billion, or 8.6 percent of the gross national product, was spent on health care in the fiscal year ending June 30, 1976. A family of four spends an average of $2600 each year for health care. Hospital costs per day have risen from less than $16 in 1950 to between $154 and $175 in 1976.[2]

More ominous than these figures, however, is the conviction of observers that the demand for medical services may be insatiable and that this will lead to continuing increases in cost. Medical economists have

[1] *Health Care in the United States,* Department of Health, Education, and Welfare, Washington, D.C., 1975, p. 7.

[2] *U.S. News and World Report,* March 28, 1977, vol. 82, no. 12, pp. 36–37.

expressed concern that we are faced with a potentially infinite demand in the face of finite resources. This demand originates not just with the consumer, but with the physician as well, and if it continues to increase it may lead to allocating resources.

A mystique seems to have developed around medical technology. Owing to new drugs, sophisticated surgical procedures, and the complex hardware found in intensive care units, patients and doctors alike appear to expect that aches and pains need not be tolerated any longer. Sometimes it appears that even death should not be tolerated. Medical advances, however, have certainly not lit up the Stygian darkness. The life expectancy of those reaching thirty years of age did not increase appreciably from the 1920s through 1973 in spite of the advances in medicine, and the increase in life expectancy since 1973 has been attributed to changes in living patterns rather than to technological advances. Medical advances certainly have great value, but their misuse due to an unwillingness to admit human mortality is costly and regressive.

This has not been emphasized adequately in the education of physicians or of the general public. Even if it had been, however, there would still be pressures to overuse the technology. Sometimes physicians do not have enough confidence in their clinical data (from their examination of the patient) and they rely excessively on sophisticated technology as a diagnostic aid. Or physicians may not correctly estimate the risk/benefit ratio before deciding on treatment. There is also a tendency for physicians to overuse technology in order to protect themselves against possible malpractice suits.

Overuse of technology increases health care costs directly. Everyone knows this. What is less well known is that it may have a far more drastic indirect effect. Not all diagnostic aids or therapeutic measures are completely safe. Many of them lead to further disability as a complication of the test or treatment. Such disabilities are called iatrogenic (physician-induced). They lead to further use of resources to deal with problems that did not exist until the patient visited the doctor.

Cost can be increased even more because of the error rate intrinsic to almost all diagnostic laboratory tests and procedures. The error rate varies from test to test, but it is rarely less than 5 percent and may be much higher. Thus, there will always be a certain number of false positive results, which show the presence of a disease that the patient does not have. More tests are then required and the cost to the patient escalates. A competent physician can reduce the number of false positive results in a variety of ways.

It is possible that medical costs could be contained or reduced if physicians and patients did not expect so much of medicine. There is not a pill for every discomfort, nor is there a corrective therapy for every disability.

Another criticism leveled at the medical profession is that the physician dehumanizes patients. The physician may be more interested in basic processes, the biological aspects of patient care, than in the patient or in the effect on the patient's life. American physicians are more skilled in handling basic disease processes now than at any time in the past, but this has come at the expense of a concern for many other aspects of the patient's life.

This is a subtle criticism, one that really cannot be confirmed or denied. What is important is that many patients feel that physicians are reluctant to accept responsibility for dealing with a disability until they can clearly demonstrate that it is due to a disease process. Beyond that, patients are sometimes concerned that, if they are ill, the doctor may initiate extensive diagnostic procedures and therapeutic regimens without adequately considering cost (risk to life, risk of further suffering, and monetary cost). The perception that physicians are unwilling or unable to deal with a patient who is somehow disabled and may or may not have an organic problem has created considerable hostility. This has led to much of the public scrutiny of the medical profession.

A variety of solutions to these problems have been suggested. Ivan Illich said that many of the problems of modern health care are related to the overuse of medical technology. One of his suggested solutions was to dispense with all licensing and legal standards.[3] Others would impose rigid regulations on medical practice. Another suggestion was that the patient's first contact with the health care system should be through a physician substitute or a less well-educated physician.[4]

We should be concerned with some of these suggestions because they may cause regression to an earlier state of American medicine in which there were almost no standards for the education of physicians. Each new medical advance brings risks and benefits, and modern patient care has become too complex to be left in the hands of less well-educated physicians or physician substitutes. Nor should we impose rigid regulations on physicians because modern medical problems are complex. At the other extreme, Illich's suggestion that all health care be deregulated invites disaster.

What the profession needs is a new emphasis on the conceptual aspects of patient care. These include skills in acquiring data, interpreting them, integrating various kinds of data, making decisions, and implementing them. Physicians who have acquired these skills should be given the authority to be the primary decision makers for their

[3] Ivan Illich, *Medical Nemesis, the Expropriation of Health*, Pantheon Books (Random House), New York, 1976.

[4] Samuel Proger, "The Education of Different Types of Physicians for Different Types of Health Care," *The Pharos*, April 1972, pp. 53-66.

patients. They would, of course, have to accept responsibility for their decisions. This is one way for the medical profession to begin to cope with change. It is probable that the development of physicians of this sort would improve quality of care at sufficiently reduced cost to make the need for other changes less urgent.

Above all, the public should be wary of simplistic or opportunistic solutions to the problems facing medicine today. This book, by defining the physician's function, demonstrates why such solutions cannot work. More effective physicians, however, could be the answer people have been seeking.

The Changing Physician Model ______ 3

Surely, if ever there was a profession in which the practitioners should constantly be thinking, observing, puzzling, and reasoning, it should be medicine.

Walter Alvarez, *The Incurable Physician*

The critical state of affairs facing the medical profession may be the most serious in its history. It involves definition of the role of physicians, education of physicians, and public trust. The very foundation of the medical profession is being rocked from within and without as people seek solutions to pressing problems.

A key factor leading to the present crisis in patient care has been the inability to determine whether modern medicine is primarily a technological discipline or a conceptual one. It is really neither. It is a conceptual science that utilizes technology when appropriate. The physician, specifically the primary physician, must be a conceptualizer if technology is to be used prudently. The technological advances of medicine, which are frequently quite dramatic, have been publicized by the media, while the conceptual aspects of the physician's function have not been sufficiently appreciated by either the medical profession or the public during the past several decades.

This situation is due, in part, to an incomplete interpretation of a report by Abraham Flexner, a lay educator who surveyed medical education in the United

States and Canada at the turn of the century.[1] He was commissioned by the Carnegie Foundation to determine how American medicine could be improved (it was in bad shape then). He completed his study with the assistance of the American Medical Association and the cooperation of the 155 medical schools he visited. He inspected classrooms, laboratories, surgeries, and clinics in those schools and issued his report in 1910.

The problems that led to the Flexner report were quite different from the problems American medicine faces today. At that time, the major problem was the quality of physicians; medical education was so poorly monitored that there was an excess of poorly educated physicians. Small communities were not complaining, as they do today, that they did not have enough doctors; instead, they complained that they had too many doctors and that few of them were prepared for medical practice. The public understood the problem.

Even before Flexner came on the scene, certain members of the medical profession had also been aware of these deficiencies. Sir William Osler, a leading medical educator of the time, pointed out the same deficiencies emphasized in the Flexner report in a lecture at the University of Minnesota in 1892.[2] He also indicated that a handful of medical educators had been engaging in an uphill fight for at least the previous 25 years. It took the Flexner report, however, to have a direct impact on this problem.

The report led to the closing of proprietary medical schools (schools run by self-styled faculties for fun and profit) and the merger of some medical schools with

[1] Abraham Flexner, *Medical Education in the United States and Canada*, Science and Health Publications, Washington, D.C., 1910.

[2] Sir William Osler, *Aequanimitas and Other Addresses*, 3d ed., Blakiston Co., Philadelphia, 1932, p. 23.

stronger ones affiliated with universities. Medical schools began to accept only students with some college education (previously some physicians had not even completed high school), and the association with universities generally improved the level of medical education. These reforms led to the development of today's medical education in a university setting adequately supplied with laboratories and with a faculty capable of doing research in the basic medical sciences.

The present scientific excellence of modern medicine was made possible by these reforms. Basic scientific knowledge was emphasized, basic research was performed in the teaching hospitals, and much was learned about disease processes because of this focus.

Flexner also stressed a second function of physicians in addition to knowing basic scientific, disease-oriented medicine:

> So far we have spoken explicitly of the fundamental sciences only. They furnish, indeed, the essential instrumental basis of medical education. *But the instrumental minimum can hardly serve as the permanent professional minimum.* It is even instrumentally inadequate. The practitioner deals with facts of two categories. Chemistry, physics, biology, enable him to apprehend one set; *he needs a different apperceptive and appreciative apparatus to deal with the other, more subtle elements. Specific preparation in this direction is much more difficult*; one must rely for the requisite insight and sympathy on a varied and enlarging cultural experience. Such enlargement of the physician's horizon is otherwise important, for scientific progress has greatly modified his ethical responsibility. His relationship was formerly to his patient—at most to his patient's family; and it was almost altogether remedial. The patient has something the matter with him; the doctor was called in to cure it. Payment of a fee ended the transaction. *But the physician's function is fast becoming social and preventive, rather than individual and curative. Upon him society relies to*

> *ascertain, and through measures essentially educational to enforce, the conditions that prevent disease and make positively for physical and moral well-being. It goes without saying that this type of doctor is first of all an educated man.*[3] [emphasis added]

Flexner said that the physician should have two functions. The first was medical, to treat disease. The second was a social function, to accept responsibility for the *total* patient and to help maintain a healthy population. He could not have foreseen the technological advances after World War II or the fragmentation of medicine into specialties. He could not have predicted the rising costs, the lack of availability of physicians, or the depersonalization of patients. But while he undoubtedly anticipated that medicine would retain the strengths outlined in his report, he was wise enough to see that a physician had to do more than treat disease. Despite his warning, however, the social function has gradually been forgotten since World War II and is only now being recalled.

The model proposed by Flexner proved useful as long as a single physician could serve both functions. These were performed by the wise and compassionate general practitioner of the past who had been educated well enough to be a "safe doctor." But in the last several decades, with the development of increasingly sophisticated forms of medical technology and the resulting development of specialties, subspecialties and superspecialties, other physician models began to appear. It frequently took only the development of a new, sophisticated tool or surgical procedure to enable some specialties to develop. Physicians in these areas were professionals who knew how to use these sophisticated

[3] Abraham Flexner, *Medical Education in the United States and Canada*, p. 26.

tools, but often did not need to know much about the total patient.

In this way, physicians began to fill distinct and separate roles after World War II instead of the single role that predominated previously. These multiple roles made it more difficult for the public and the medical profession to pinpoint the function of the physician. Rosemary Stevens suggests this in the closing of her book *American Medicine and the Public Interest*:

> Evaluating the intellectuality of medical education, length of curriculum, selection of students, encouragement of multiple track teaching systems, and forms of graduate medical education is still largely the preserve of the professional institutions of medicine. *At root these are questions of what, indeed, is a physician? And this question is as yet unanswered.*[4] [emphasis added]

Isn't this a curious fact? Isn't it time to examine the significance of the fact that the role and function of the modern physician are unclear to both society and the medical profession? Isn't it also time to see whether definition is attainable?

Physicians, of course, take care of sick people and try to prevent illness. But ask physicians or the public what physicians do, and their answers will demonstrate the fragmentation of modern medicine. Physicians examine and make diagnoses, take X-rays, look through microscopes, prescribe treatments, look in various body orifices. They counsel and advise, set broken bones, conduct basic research. They deliver babies and check on their develop-

[4] Rosemary Stevens, *American Medicine and the Public Interest*, Yale University Press, New Haven, Connecticut, 1971, p. 531.

ment. They perform operations. A physician runs a company's medical department.

None of these duties adequately describes the function of physicians, and neither do the situations described in the media, where it is more a question of dramatic contrast than routine. News reports tell of doctors who have discovered and used new drugs and surgical procedures, while television drama presents physicians who are involved in tense situations that are often solved by complex technology. To attract the public attention, life-death, happiness-unhappiness, mental health-psychosis situations are required. But the technology presented only awes the public; the result is a public that knows nothing of a physician's function.

Since the Flexner report, research, technology, and specialization have been increasingly emphasized in medical education. Although this solved the problems that existed at the turn of the century, it is also responsible for the current problems caused by lack of appreciation of the social role of the physician. Where should a physician who fills this role be in the medical hierarchy? How much authority should such a physician be given? With advances in medical technology, the practice of medical specialties has increased in stature and in volume. The increase came at the expense of diminishing the influence of the generalist, particularly the general practitioner, in medical education and patient care. It need only be pointed out that in the 1930s, 85 percent of the graduating medical students entered general practice directly after internship, but by the late 1960s, 85 percent of the graduating seniors had committed themselves to a career in one of the specialties.

This trend reached the point in the 1950s and 1960s where people said that general practice was dead. This statement was sometimes made by members of various factions within the medical profession who were involved in intraprofessional rivalry, but it was also made by many thoughtful physicians who were reviewing the possible role of the general practitioner in a technological environment. It was becoming apparent that the half-life of any physician's biomedical knowledge was becoming progressively shorter, and that it would be necessary to specialize in order to make this demand on continuing education manageable. Right now, the half-life of a physician's basic medical knowledge is approximately five years. That is, half of a physician's knowledge about the biochemical processes of the body and about the diagnosis and treatment of disease changes within five years—the information is amplified, linked with other information, or shown to be in error.

The physician must constantly keep up with new knowledge and advances. So when one looks at the historical role of the general practitioner, who was active in all specialties and used selected forms of technology from each, the hopelessness of keeping up with advances in all fields becomes apparent.

Awareness of this difficulty influenced medical students to avoid general practice in the years after World War II. The graduating class of the University of Minnesota Medical School in 1945 was its first in which half the seniors chose a specialty career. In addition, more and more general practitioners gave up their practices and went into medical specialties, even ten or twenty years after they had entered general practice. Physicians who left it rarely entered any of the broad patient care specialties such as internal medicine or pediatrics. Instead, they chose the more technologically oriented specialties such as radiology, laboratory medicine, ophthalmology, anesthesiology, and pathology. This further removed them from participation in total patient care.

The division of the broadest medical specialties, internal medicine and pediatrics, into subspecialties such as hematology, gastroenterology, and endocrinology also occurred during this period. In the 1940s, medical residents in internal medicine and pediatrics could choose to devote the bulk of their careers to caring for the total patient. By the late 1960s, many residents were choosing residency programs in subspecialties with the intention of limiting their practices to a single organ system.

Technological advances in the subspecialties encouraged this trend, but the role models provided by teachers were also a contributing factor. In most medical schools and teaching hospitals, there was a drastic decline in the number of physicians who practiced broad, clinical medicine. The students could not help but believe that the body of knowledge that a general clinician must possess was so vast that it was unencompassable and that they must enter a narrow specialty to survive in medical practice.

These changes had a far-reaching effect on patient care. The concept seemed to be accepted, without ever being articulated, that the physician need not be concerned with the total patient. The subspecialty trainee was being taught patient care in the context of a single organ system and its diseases. The patient who had a problem that one physician could not solve could be sent to a specialist down the hall. This was the example set in teaching hospitals, where students were shown that the patient was their responsibility only when the symptoms fit their specialty, and then only for as long as the patient was in their hospital.

Attending staff in these hospitals did not have any further responsibility for the care of patients after they left the hospital and returned to their own physicians. Because of this, physicians trained in the 1950s and 1960s were not exposed to the skills of providing total patient care for any period, because the opportunities were not available in the teaching hospitals. When one considers that, in a typical population, 72 percent visit a physician in a clinic at least once a year, 10 percent are admitted to a hospital at least once a year, and only 1 percent are admitted to a university hospital at least once a year, it becomes obvious that medical students are not receiving an education based on the overall needs of the public.[5]

With fewer physicians becoming available to the public for broad patient care, studies were commissioned in the early and middle 1960s to determine the cause of this phenomenon and to suggest how to reverse the trend. The Millis report, commissioned by the American Medical Association and chaired by John S. Millis, then president of Western Reserve University, is the best known.[6] The commission that prepared it coined the phrase "primary physician." The report recommended that programs in graduate medical education be revised to educate a new kind of physician with a new body of knowledge for total patient care. This physician would accept primary responsibility for the patient's welfare on a continuing and comprehensive basis and would be the patient's first contact and point of entry into the health care system. The commission also said that the primary physician's responsibility for the patient should remain even when the services of other medical specialties are required.

The report indicated three major reasons for the failure to develop substantial numbers of these physicians:

> 1. General practice, once the mainstay of medicine, has gradually lost prestige as the specialties have risen in honor and accomplishments. In deciding upon his own career, the young physician may never see excellent examples of comprehensive, continuing care or highly qualified and prestigious primary physicians. He is certain, however, to see a

[5] Kerr L. White, "Life and Death in Medicine," *Scientific American*, September 1973, vol. 229, pp. 23–33.

[6] *The Report of the Citizens Commission on Graduate Medical Education*, Council on Medical Education, American Medical Association, 1966.

variety of specialists and to observe that they usually enjoy higher prestige, greater hospital privileges, and more favorable working conditions than do general practitioners.

2. Educational opportunities that would serve to interest students in family practice and provide interns and residents with appropriate training are few in number and often poorer in quality than the programs leading to the specialties.

3. The conditions of practice for a general practitioner or a physician interested in family practice are thought to be less attractive than the conditions and privileges enjoyed by specialists.[7]

Most significantly, the commission then wrote, "*All three of these difficulties can be overcome, but heroic work will be required. It is time for a revolution, not a few patchwork adaptations*"[7] [emphasis added].

Since the report was released, agreement has been reached that practitioners of general internal medicine, family medicine, and pediatrics fulfill the role of the primary physician. These are the specialties that are most readily adapted to total and continuing responsibility for the patient. But the report was released at a time when generalists and specialists were vying for higher status in patient care, and this internal rivalry obscured some of the points of the report.

The dispute has confused people because partisans involved in it were suggesting that they were the only primary physicians. The general practitioner became identified with the primary physician in the public mind, but because of the functional demands on the modern physician, the two terms are no longer synonomous. In

[7] *The Report of the Citizens Commission on Graduate Medical Education*, p. 38.

fact, the generalist of today (the primary physician) is a specialist in a well-defined area.

The problem could be clarified if we better understood the function of the physician. We would then know how the primary physician fits into the medical hierarchy. We stated earlier that the primary physician is a conceptualizer who uses technology prudently. What is important about this statement is that the physician's judgment is taken for granted.

We also said earlier that decision making is the major challenge in medicine today. The physician most directly responsible for the ongoing care of the patient must be given authority to implement the decisions commensurate with the responsibility assumed in making them. However, before American medicine and the American public can deal with those matters, it must face the question raised by Rosemary Stevens: "What, indeed, is a physician?"

Two distinct types of physicians should be available: conceptually oriented physicians and technologically oriented physicians. Each type is indispensable to the public. The conceptually oriented physicians would be the physicians of first contact, and their practice would be based on primary responsibility for long-term continuing care of a patient. Most of their practice would be conducted in their offices, although they would use hospitals and technologically oriented physicians when necessary. The technologically oriented physicians would be those who usually limit their practice to either an organ system, such as the digestive or circulatory system, or a procedure, such as certain kinds of surgical procedures. Others would limit their work to certain types of technology such as X-ray or anesthesia. The nature of their practice often demands the use of extremely sophisticated, invasive, and sometimes dangerous forms of technology. Their practice is mainly consultative, limited to a single disease process in any particular patient, and much, if not most, of their work is performed in hospitals.

Both kinds of physicians are important for patient care. The conceptually oriented (primary) physician would have extreme difficulty conducting a daily practice were it not for the impressive array of modern equipment at the technologically oriented physician's command. The problem, however, is that the technologically oriented physicians have gained considerable stature and recognition from the public at large and from their colleagues, while the conceptually oriented physicians have fared less well. This has led to progressively smaller numbers of medical students choosing to be primary physicians.

Sir William Osler once referred to the internist as the "pure physician." It must be remembered that in Osler's time, pediatrics had not developed as a separate specialty, and Osler was, in today's terms, an internist and pediatrician (a primary physician). The following excerpt from a talk he delivered to the New York Academy of Medicine in 1897 is equally applicable today:

> It was with the greatest pleasure that I accepted an invitation to address this section of the Academy on the importance of internal medicine as a vocation. I wish there were another term to designate the wide field of medical practice which remains after the separation of surgery, midwifery, and gynecology. Not itself a specialty (though it embraces at least half a dozen), its cultivators cannot be called specialists, but bear without reproach the good old name physician, in contradistinction to general practitioner, surgeons, obstetricians, and gynecologists. I have heard the fear expressed that in this country the sphere of the physician proper is becoming more and more restricted, and perhaps this is true; but I maintain (and I hope to convince you) that the opportunities are still great, that the harvest truly is plenteous, and that the labourers scarcely sufficient to meet the demand. At the outset I would like to emphasize the fact

> that the student of internal medicine cannot be a specialist. The manifestations of almost any one of the important diseases in the course of a few years will "box the compass" of the specialties.[8]

Perhaps the question "What is a physician?" should be rephrased to read "What is a primary physician?" For if the role and function of the primary physician could be identified and agreed on by the public and the medical profession, and if sufficient numbers of them could be educated, we would have come a long way toward resolving the problems facing American medicine. There is now a general lack of understanding of the responsibilities of the primary physician. Until they can be defined and understood and until corresponding authority is provided, there will continue to be a shortage of primary physicians.

This book is directed to the general public because in the next several years the public will have to make some major decisions about the future direction of patient care in the United States. It is imperative that the role and function of the primary physician become widely known if these are to be rational decisions. Flexner said something similar in his report:

> The striking and significant facts which are here brought out are of enormous consequence not only to the medical practitioner, but to every citizen of the United States and Canada; for it is a singular fact that the organization of medical education in this country has hitherto been such as not only to commercialize the process of education itself, but also to obscure in the minds of the public any discrimination between the well-trained physician and the physician who has had no adequate training whatsoever. As a rule, Americans, when they avail themselves of the services of a physician, make only the slightest inquiry as to what his

[8] Sir William Osler, *Aequanimitas and Other Addresses*, p. 133.

> previous training and preparation have been. One of the problems of the future is to educate the public itself to appreciate the fact that very seldom, under existing conditions, does a patient receive the best aid which it is possible to give him in the present state of medicine, and that is due mainly to the fact that a vast army of men is admitted to the practice of medicine who are untrained in sciences fundamental to the profession and quite without a sufficient experience with disease. A right education of public opinion is one of the problems of future medical education.[9]

It must be emphasized that the problems were different in Flexner's time. The crisis then was one of quality of medical education. This is not true today. The basic preparation of the student physician is not in question at present. What is in question is the definition of the function of the two kinds of physicians and the establishment of proper educational programs to prepare the conceptually oriented (primary) physicians for their future tasks.

[9] Abraham Flexner, *Medical Education in the United States and Canada*, p. 10.

Influence of Technology on Medical Education — 4

The reductionist approach has been immensely fruitful in discoveries and has made it possible to convert certain aspects of knowledge into power. Unfortunately, it has resulted in the neglect of many important fields of science and has encouraged an attitude toward nature which is socially destructive in the long run. The study of the interplay *between the component parts of the system is at least as important as the study of any or all of the isolated components.*

Rene Dubos, *So Human an Animal*

When Flexner's recommendations were implemented, basic sciences were emphasized. Medical schools and teaching hospitals built and staffed laboratories to teach science and to develop the students' skills in the treatment of disease. Full-time faculty members were appointed to teach basic sciences and were encouraged to do research as well. Some physicians practicing in the community became part-time members of the medical school faculty to teach clinical medicine, but they eventually relinquished their role as community physicians to serve as full-time faculty members within the university hospitals. They became consultants and researchers as well as teachers, and their research was mostly limited to a specific area of basic medical science.

The research function of the faculty assumed greater importance and became more time-consuming. As the kind and amount of research became a primary factor in promotions, the statement "publish or perish" acquired more meaning in medical schools. Indeed, it has been said facetiously that publications are useful criteria for evaluating faculty because "you can weigh them, you can measure them, you can count them, and, if worse comes to worst, you can even read them."

Faculty clinicians who retained a general interest in broad medical practice—the primary or conceptually oriented physicians—were gradually lost in this process. Technologically oriented physicians, who view medicine as an exact science, began to dominate medical education. The philosophy taught was that the primary concern of the physician should be the eradication of any organic disease that may be present. The corollary to this, of course, was that if a well-defined disease process could not be found, the patient was no longer the physician's responsibility. From this time on there was a decline in the stature and influence of the clinician with broad interests in medical education.

Soon most teachers of medical students were spending more time on basic research than on patient care. Equally significantly, the nature of that research changed as medical technology became more sophisticated. Whereas much of early medical research was clinical (groups of patients treated in different ways and compared to each other), much of current medical research is laboratory research.

This has led to the many brilliant discoveries in medical science of the past several decades. But the education of the medical students has suffered in the process. In the past, they had been taught by broad clinicians and learned many of the subtleties of patient care from them. For the last several decades, however, teachers have been primarily researchers. Students have always viewed medical practice through their teachers' eyes, so now the concepts of basic medical research are the concepts students associate with patient care. But these concepts are not applicable in clinical practice. The laboratory researcher, for example, tries to control all the variables of an experiment except one (and frequently is successful in doing this). The medical practitioner, on the other hand, has to make diagnostic and therapeutic decisions in a limited time and in the face of considerable uncertainty and continuing change in the patient's behavioral and physical status.

One of the factors that helped establish this trend was the changing experiential background of the medical school faculty. Previously, faculty members were recruited from outstanding community clinicians, but after World War II, young physicians were recruited directly from the graduate ranks. This resulted in a faculty with no patient care experience outside the medical schools and university hospitals.

Medical students must have inferred that patient care could be conducted with the same rigid controls that are part of a formal scientific experiment. There was no way for them to know that the population of patients in a university hospital had totally different characteristics from the population of patients in the community. Again, the technologically oriented physician assumed a position of dominance over the conceptually oriented physician.

This is, however, not an either/or situation, in which one of the two factions must succeed and the other fail. Obviously both types of physicians are necessary for exemplary patient care, but developments in the past several decades have had the result that the primary physician does not fit well into the present hierarchical structure of medical education and medical practice. What we are talking about here is the nature of Thomas Kuhn's scientific revolutions—a new paradigm, in which the primary physician's judgment dominates, must be introduced.[1] But a new paradigm will always threaten those who have much invested in the old paradigm.

This revolution resolves itself into the question of which type of approach to problem solving should be used: the Cartesian or the configuration approach. The Cartesian approach requires reducing the problem to the smallest possible dimension and attempting to solve it at that level. In patient care, this has led to the simplification of the total organism, first by division into body and mind and then by division into organ systems, enzyme systems, cells, and even cellular components. The configuration approach, described by Peter Drucker, involves viewing problems in the context of total patterns.[2] In medicine, this means that all of the patient's problems must be evaluated along with the immediate complaint before a decision is made. An example of each approach was given in Chapter 1; the decision to restore the circulation surgically was based on the Cartesian approach and the decision to amputate immediately on the configuration approach.

In the old paradigm, disease is the sine qua non of patient care; that is, in the absence of a defined organic problem, the patient is considered healthy. The patient is not the responsibility of the physician even though he or she does not feel well. Consequently, the education of the medical student has been largely limited to those facts necessary to understand disease.

In the new paradigm, however, disease is not the sine qua non. A primary physician recognizes that a patient can have both a disease and symptoms, but that the symptoms may be unrelated to the disease. The physician also

[1] Thomas S. Kuhn, *The Structure of Scientific Revolutions*, 2d ed., University of Chicago Press, Chicago, 1962.

[2] Peter Drucker, *Age of Discontinuity*, Harper & Row, New York, 1969.

recognizes that a patient may have disabling symptoms in the absence of any disease and that this situation must also be dealt with. The total pattern must be defined by the physician, who should then act appropriately.

Kuhn used the term paradigm because scientific theory is constantly changing to better fit new discoveries and new explanations. What is accepted as scientific truth is really only a model or a view that helps one understand the world. In patient care, the Cartesian approach has been the dominant paradigm. It has been highly successful in the history of science for several centuries, but strict adherence to it in medical practice is now leading to many of the current problems in patient care.

The dominance of the Cartesian approach is understandable when one views the impressive technological advances since World War II. Artificial life support systems, coronary artery bypass surgery, organ transplantation, and advances in the treatment of cancer and of various forms of endocrine and infectious diseases are some examples of these advances. Newer forms of contraception are further examples. These advances were so brilliant that, for a time, nearly everyone thought that all medical problems could be resolved by the application of rigid scientific principles. Even today, many members of the medical profession and the general public believe this, although their numbers are diminishing. Yet strict adherence to this paradigm leads to many problems, such as the tragedies associated with the inappropriate use of artificial life support systems.

What has happened is that the guidance system has lagged behind the technology. The configuration approach must serve as the guidance system for the Cartesian approach. The question of whether a specific form of technology should be used must always be asked—and answered. The answer often requires keen judgment and is based on careful examination of the patient's total situation. Physicians trained exclusively in the Cartesian approach to problem solving are not usually prepared to make such an analysis. It requires conceptual skills to decide what provides the patient with the best chance of being helped and the least chance of being hurt. Such decisions are difficult and require both confidence and courage.

All physicians need to have a knowledge of both approaches to problem solving, but the primary care of the patient should be directed by a broadly trained clinician who is able to make accurate decisions about the use of sophisticated equipment. Abraham Maslow and others have described a similar conflict between the behaviorists and phenomenologists in psychology.[3,4] As Maslow said, "If the only tool you have is a hammer, everything looks like a nail." This is true in medical practice too; that is, a hammer is effective if you want to drive a nail into a piece of wood, but no one would use it to pin a note to a bulletin board. Since primary physicians are not committed to any particular area of technology, they are in a position to be most objective in deciding whether to use various diagnostic and therapeutic devices.

For many years, this conceptual basis of patient care was dealt with summarily by saying that it was the "art of medicine." It was felt, and still is for the most part, that the physician either brought these skills along to medical school or developed them experientially. Since they were not considered teachable, physicians had to acquire them by themselves.

These are not intuitive skills; they are comprised of a number of previously undefined components from other

[3] Abraham Maslow, *The Psychology of Science*, Harper & Row, New York, 1966.

[4] William D. Hitt, "Two Models of Man," *American Psychologist*, July 1969, vol. 24, p. 651.

scholarly disciplines such as psychology, sociology, communications, statistics, logic, and so on. They can now be defined and taught, and one can take the position that, just as the lack of knowledge of medical advances results in a poor physician, inadequate development of conceptual skills has the same result. These skills consist of the ability of the physician to elicit accurate and complete data from the patient, to interpret the data and evaluate their significance, to relate these data to a strong background of medical knowledge, and to make reasonable decisions and implement them.

If all physicians had been taught these skills, today's crisis in patient care would probably not exist. On the other hand, if there were no physicians trained in research and the use of various forms of technology, we would probably be faced with a different kind of crisis. It is really a question of balance, of how to use the various kinds of physicians. It is also a question of how to allocate authority commensurate with the responsibility each kind of physician assumes in various clinical settings. Technologically oriented physicians have tools at their disposal, but since they have not been adequately prepared for total patient care, they are not always able to judge objectively whether the best interests of the patient are served by using those tools. Because of the prevailing tendency to reduce problems to simpler levels, the general public and physicians have unrealistically high expectations of technology. When one tries to explain human suffering on the basis of malfunction of a single organ system, there is frequently a tendency to view cure as being fairly simple to achieve. The price to the patient, however, is often higher than orginally estimated.

It used to be said that there is a modest advantage to the public in being served by a competent physician rather than no physician at all, but that there is a tremendous disadvantage to being served by an incompetent physician rather than no physician at all. That idea was conceived before diagnostic and therapeutic technology were as far advanced as they are now, but it arose from similar considerations. It was another way of saying, "First of all, do no harm."

Why Seek Medical Help? 5

During the present century, one of the most striking internal trends in medical sciences has been the partial return to a generalized pathology.

Richard H. Shryock, *Medicine in America, Historical Essays*

Patients do not go to physicians expecting the treatment to be worse than the disease; yet a major problem in patient care is that this sometimes is the case, many times needlessly so. This is due to several factors, one of which, the dominance of technology and research in many of the teaching hospitals, has already been discussed. Other more subtle reasons are related to the cultural attitudes of health professionals and the public toward sickness. These attitudes may reduce the objectivity of physicians toward patients' problems. This, in turn, may lead physicians to impose their own values on patients without even realizing it.

Sociologists have done most of the research that describes these attitudes toward sickness behavior, and their approach is interesting and useful. They define sickness behavior as deviant (deviant behavior is a variant from the cultural norm). Sickness and criminal deviance are the only two major types of deviant behavior recognized. These two types, however, are not sharply defined, and certain types of behavior may be classified as one or the other at different times. For instance, chemical addiction used to be considered criminally deviant, but it is now usually considered a form of sickness deviance. Another example is psychiatric illness, certain forms of which are sometimes considered criminal deviance and other times sickness deviance.

David Mechanic describes sickness deviance in greater detail, dividing it into a "medical model" and a "psychiatric model."[1] The medical model is represented by clearly defined disease processes which have decisive diagnostic criteria and clear-cut natural histories and for which specific and often successful forms of treatment are available. This model enables the physician to make a precise diagnosis of an illness, to define the outcome if it were left untreated, and to advise the patient what to expect from treatment. Bacterial infections, for which specific antibiotics are available; acute appendicitis, for which a surgical procedure exists; and hypothyroidism, for which specific replacement therapy is available, are examples of diseases that fit this model.

In the psychiatric model, the diagnostic criteria are considerably less precise. Whereas a majority of physicians can study the data and come to the same conclusions for a disease that fits the medical model, illnesses in the psychiatric model are less clear-cut and physicians frequently disagree on diagnosis, treatment, and prognosis. This is true not only of the obvious diseases in this model such as schizophrenia and paranoia, but also of the many functional disabilities of patients caused by emotional strain associated with daily living patterns. It is particularly true of emotionally induced disability occurring in patients with knowledge of coexisting serious illness. In fact, symptomatic problems and their attendant functional disabilities

[1] David Mechanic, *Medical Sociology*, The Free Press, New York, 1968, chap. 3.

caused by emotional strain account for 50 to 75 percent of daily medical practice.

Physicians are generally more uncomfortable with problems that fit the psychiatric model, partly because their medical education emphasized the medical model, and partly because of societal attitudes toward illness. When patients adopt the sick role and visit a physician, sociologists say that they assume new responsibilities and privileges. The responsibilities are that the patients are expected to want to recover from their illness, and that they will do whatever is necessary to effect recovery. The privileges are that the patients are temporarily relieved of their other responsibilities and that they are not considered responsible for their condition. Physicians have trouble with this definition of the sick role in patients with emotionally induced disability, probably because the sick role was defined in terms of acute, well-defined organic disease. All four criteria of the sick role clearly apply to the medical model, but they do not fit the psychiatric model as well.

This is important in patient care, because a great amount of chronic disability results from emotional strain. Sometimes the strain is caused by the patient's realization that the disease is incurable, while at other times it originates in the patient's socioeconomic environment in the total absence of organic disease. Particularly in the latter case, when the patient is experiencing symptoms and may be disabled despite the absence of disease, the concept of the sick role may cause a dilemma for physicians because of the societal attitudes they have accepted. They may be suspicious that the patient does not want to become well or that the patient has somehow caused the disability. It becomes quite difficult for physicians to retain their objectivity toward the patient if they begin to think this way, and the result may be that the patient is rejected.

Another problem is that physicians now see a great deal

of chronic disability resulting from the residua of a variety of organic diseases that formerly caused death but that can now be controlled for some time. For example, some forms of heart disease, diabetes mellitus, and cancer can now be controlled for years, whereas they used to cause death in a relatively short time. Some of these diseases lead to a certain amount of disability that is not correctable.

The concept of the sick role creates a problem in the latter situations because of the responsibilities the sick role places on the patient. The patient is expected to want to recover and to do whatever is necessary to recover. This may lead to unrealistic expectations of the patient and the physician, which in turn lead to overutilization of diagnostic and therapeutic resources. In many of these situations, the risks of the tests and/or treatment far exceed the small chance of benefit to the patient.

An individual patient will seek a physician because, in the simplest form, the patient has a question and wants it answered. This is probably the common denominator in the decisions of most individuals to become patients, but the background activities that lead to the question will vary considerably from one segment of society to another. For example, it has been shown that some ethnic groups within American society respond to pain stimuli simply with an intense desire to relieve themselves of the pain; so this desire will lead them to become patients. Other groups feel little concern over the discomfort itself, but they become quite concerned about the possible underlying causes of the pain, and this concern will lead them to physicians.

There is also variation in how the decision to become a patient is made among the socioeconomic strata of society. The middle and upper classes respond more rapidly to symptoms of disability by seeking medical advice, because, it is thought, they are better educated in health maintenance. They have been taught and believe that early intervention in a situation of this sort can minimize or eliminate subsequent disability. On the other hand, the lower middle class and the most disadvantaged classes are more likely to view their bodies as they would a machine. They believe that their bodies have a certain useful life and that they should continue to use them until they wear out.[2] Part of the reason for this behavior is their lack of access to physicians and the high cost of medical care, but an important reason is that they have not been educated in the value of health maintenance.

There are also some other factors that complicate the decision to become a patient. Some individuals, on feeling ill, will first seek advice from nonmedical sources, such as family, neighbors, and friends. Or they may seek other health providers such as folk practitioners or cultists of various types and resort to a physician only if these efforts fail. There is also a tendency for some people to deny illness, hoping that whatever troubles them will just go away. It may reach the point where their employers send them to a physician. Denial is not always a problem, because sometimes the patient has had previous experience with the symptom and realizes that it will clear up soon, but at the other extreme, denial can be catastrophic. Studies of patients who had chest pains associated with heart attacks and who deferred seeking medical advice during the critical initial period show that many of these patients died from the attack before they could receive definitive care.

If physicians are to gain maximum information from a patient, they must understand that there are a variety of paths that a patient may follow before consulting them. They must obtain and understand the behavioral data as well as the

[2] Anselm L. Strauss, "Medical Organization, Medical Care, and Lower Income Groups," *Social Science and Medicine,* 1969, vol. 3, pp. 143–177.

biomedical data if they are to understand what their patient's questions are.

The patient may not state a question clearly; this is one of the difficulties associated with daily patient care. If the patient's primary question—the reason for being in the physician's office—is not answered by the physician, the patient will frequently feel that the visit has been useless. The patient may then seek further medical advice or fail to follow the doctor's recommendations. This will lead to further cost for that patient: the cost of duplication of effort by other physicians, or the cost of prolongation of disability caused by failure to follow recommendations.

The physician must be aware that the traditional sick role evolved from the medical model, in which organic disease could be treated with a decisive therapeutic regimen. Now that chronic disability makes up a larger proportion of patient care, physicians must be able to determine patients' questions accurately and answer them explicitly. Before this can be done, physicians must become aware of the significance of their preference for the medical model and their attitudes toward sickness behavior in patients who have symptoms without demonstrable organic problems.

These are some of the kinds of knowledge that all primary (conceptually oriented) physicians should have in order to understand patients' problems more clearly. The lack of emphasis on behavioral sciences such as medical sociology is one of the major failures of medical education. It is partly responsible for many of the current problems in patient care.

What Is Health? 6

He to whom only the outward and physical evil is laid open knoweth, oftentimes, but half the evil which he is called upon to cure. A bodily disease, which we look upon as whole and entire within itself, may, after all, be but a symptom of some ailment in the spiritual part.

Nathaniel Hawthorne, *The Scarlet Letter*

The question "What is health?" may seem simplistic, since health is something with which everyone is familar. Yet it is a concept that needs to be defined if we are to better understand the primary physician's function. People seek a physician's advice when they have questions about their health, and the physician will help them when they have problems with their health. But when do people have problems with health? These problems arise not only when someone has a well-defined disease process. More frequently, they occur without an organic cause, and physicians have difficulty treating the patient appropriately. They may tell the patient that nothing is wrong or may prescribe a drug and treat the symptoms only. In both cases, however, the physician has stopped looking for the cause of the symptoms.

This happens because most physicians behave as if they define health simply as the absence of disease. This has been and continues to be implicitly taught in medical schools; so when a patient has no detectable disease, physicians may feel that there is no immediate need for treatment. Their personal definition of health does not require them to be concerned when the patient is functionally disabled unless there is an organic cause for that disability.

That was how I was taught to view health. When I opened a medical practice, however, that definition posed problems for me. Patients with arthritis, for example, came to see me, and they frequently considered themselves healthy. So did diabetics and patients with ulcers. In fact, many patients with long-term problems such as these considered themselves to be quite healthy and happy and were living satisfying, fulfilling lives.

On the other hand, some patients would come in who were in fine physical condition, yet they were functionally disabled in some way. The disability could have been caused by a death in the family, by not getting a promotion at work, by problems with a friend or family member, but never by an organic problem. These patients, while physically sound, could not function. Under these circumstances, I began to wonder "Who is healthy?" and began to consider patients with long-term disabilities as healthy when their attitude and functional status justified it. I also began to think of patients who considered themselves unhealthy as having a problem that warranted my attention regardless of the presence or absence of demonstrable disease.

The patient's perception of health thus assumed great importance in my practice and it still does. It is certainly not the only factor to be considered in determining whether a patient is healthy, but it frequently helps a physician formulate a useful treatment plan. Instead of thinking of health as the absence of disease, I began to consider it to be a value judgment, first made by the patient but on which both the physician and the patient must ultimately agree.

Physicians must be quite perceptive if they are to use this definition to benefit their patients. They must be able to determine when a patient does not have a disease, and then also be able to determine what might be causing the patient's symptoms. Then, they must be able to use their findings in a way that will help the patient. Everyone is familiar with how physicians handle episodic disease problems. In fact, a physician who was unable to recognize and treat the common diseases to which people are susceptible would not long be considered a physician. But physicians must also be able to deal with functional disabilities that have no organic cause.

Because most of the kinds of health problems a primary physician sees (50 to 75 percent) are psychologically induced, this definition of health as a value judgment is particularly important. The patient becomes a sort of partner with the physician and thus becomes more willing to discuss and examine the problem. This makes it easier for the physician to decide what is causing the symptoms.

In many instances, patients are unwilling to accept a physician's judgment of their health. Examples of people not following a physician's advice are legion. Viewing health as a value judgment helps to resolve this problem because it forces the physician to determine the patients' perceptions of their own health. Having done that, the physician is in a better position to decide whether to agree or disagree on the basis of the clinical findings. If the physician agrees, the patient is simply advised appropriately; if the physician disagrees, it is necessary to try to alter the patient's judgment in such a way that the patient will cooperate with the recommended treatment.

For example, patients whose blood pressure is slightly elevated may judge that they are healthy because they are experiencing no symptoms and feel well. Because of this, they may be reluctant to take medication several times a day for an indefinite period. When this happens, the physician must convince the patients that they are not completely healthy. If the physician is successful, the patients will be more likely to take their medications because of their new understanding of the nature of the disease.

Conversely, patients sometimes consult a physician complaining of a specific pain for which the physician can find no organic cause. Psychophysiological bowel disease is an example of this. This can be an extremely painful disorder; its symptoms can be so severe that these patients sometimes undergo surgical exploration. There is no organic problem, however, and surgeons discover this when they operate. The causes of this problem can be any of a number of things, ranging from boredom to the presence of a fatal illness in a loved one. The threat of financial disaster may also manifest itself in this way.

The problem that this disability and others like it pose for physicians is whether the patient should be considered healthy. Physicians do not like to see these problems because there is no organic disability, as established by a careful physical examination. The question then is what to do with the patient. Should the physician dismiss the patient, saying that there is no problem and the patient is healthy? Or should the physician try to determine the psychological causes of the symptoms and attempt to treat them?

Such patients have made judgments about their health, based on the pain they feel. The physician has also made a judgment about the patient's health. The two judgments are frequently at odds, but the physician cannot help by dismissing the patient as healthy. What the physician must do is explain to the patient what has been learned and then try to counsel the patient on how to cope with whatever problems are responsible for the symptoms.

In a sense, this definition is based on the fact that the physician's authority is ultimately derived from the public.

It comes through legislative channels, with the physician being granted a license to practice when certain criteria have been fulfilled. The physician must have a diploma, which is acquired by graduation from an approved medical school, indicating that the physician has learned enough to be a "safe physician." After graduation, the physician must demonstrate again that a certain expertise has been acquired by passing tests given by a state or national board of medical examiners. A final component of licensure is that certain character references must be provided on behalf of the applicant. Only when these requirements are fulfilled is a license granted to practice medicine.

It is frequently thought that the American Medical Association grants the licenses, or that physicians are granted the privilege of practicing medicine simply because of belonging to the AMA. The AMA does not grant licenses, legislatures do, although they rely on the advice of physicians in medical matters.

The concept of health as a value judgment should remind the public that it is ultimately responsible for who is licensed. By defining health in the context of patients' perceptions of well-being, physicians become more accountable to patients. Physicians have always been responsible for how they treat the body, but now, with this definition, they must also respond to patients' perceptions. Patients cease to be passive recipients of care. This is proper, since the public mandate to the medical profession is that it restore and maintain health. Since the public grants the licenses, it has the right to expect that this mandate be fulfilled.

It is important that any definition of health that is accepted be very limited in scope; it must be one that physicians can use in clinical practice. By using a limited definition, such as the one suggested here, patients can expect more from their physicians and have those expectations satisfied. Patients will not feel as though their questions are unanswered and then seek another physician's advice, thereby duplicating efforts.

The World Health Organization has a good definition of health, but it is too inclusive to be of much use in the physician's office. It defines personal health as "a state of complete physical, mental and social well-being and not merely the absence of any disease or infirmity." This definition goes beyond the scope of what can be expected from physicians. It incorporates all the professions into a broad type of social engineering. It implies that health is an economic problem broader than the present relationship between illness and poverty, that it is a social problem of greater magnitude than the goals of national health insurance, and that it is a political problem that would bring everything to an ideal conclusion when resolved. The individual physician-patient relationship certainly falls within the scope of this definition, but this definition will not help a physician improve the quality of patient care. That is what we are attempting to improve right now.

One of the major changes in patient care in the last several decades underscores the importance of having physicians who can deal with patients' judgments concerning health. It is now possible to prolong useful life in many forms of disease, such as cancer, heart disease, or certain endocrine diseases, which used to cause death fairly soon after the onset of symptoms. When these diseases are diagnosed now, secondary symptoms frequently result because of patients' fears of terminal illnesses. I once had a patient who had a cancer removed surgically and, although there was no evidence that cancer had recurred in the years since the operation, the patient continued to have a variety of symptoms. The patient was uncertain of the success of the operation and considered himself unhealthy. Here, the value judgment manifested itself in the symptoms, something that can easily happen.

It is imperative that certain physicians—the primary

physicians—be taught the necessary skills to deal with problems of this sort. Not only do they have to deal with the secondary symptoms that patients sometimes develop along with serious diseases, but they also have to deal with symptoms in people who do not have any disease at all. The public seems to be more aware of diseases today as well as more aware of the ability of medicine to prolong life and sometimes the agony of terminal diseases. People will worry about the possibility of having these diseases; sometimes they will become so concerned that otherwise healthy persons will develop disabling symptoms. The physician initially contacted must be perceptive enough to recognize and deal with these problems. For too long, patients have been at risk of being dismissed as healthy if their physicians found no organic disease to explain their symptoms.

Defining health as a value judgment on which the physicians and patients must agree requires that physicians recognize many of these problems. If physicians could be taught to be more aware of the existence of these problems, recognition could be accomplished more quickly and with less reliance on modern diagnostic technology. It also requires that physicians develop the skills necessary to counsel these patients, and that they develop understanding, patience, and tolerance for those who do not fit rigidly into the medical model of the sick role.

Thus, realistic and attainable goals for subsequent diagnostic and therapeutic regimens can be set. When cure is possible, the necessary measures can be taken. If the patient cannot be cured, the definition permits use of whatever measures are necessary to control the disease and to comfort the patient. In cases where the symptoms are caused by emotional stresses, the physician has a working definition that will make it possible to satisfy the patients' concerns and expectations. It requires that physicians be much more than artisans or doers or users of technology.

This definition can be expanded to act as a rough guideline for health maintenance programs as well. Health maintenance programs are ones in which individuals participate and that are usually initiated through public education programs. Promotion of the use of seat belts, articles warning of the dangers of alcohol abuse, and articles demonstrating the association of cigarette smoking with lung cancer, heart disease, and chronic lung disease are examples. Individuals hear of these and may decide to modify their behavior. Preventive medicine programs are similar, but they do not usually call for individual participation. Mass immunization, fluoridation of water, and proper sewage disposal are examples of measures taken under the preventive medicine programs. These are designed to prevent mass outbreaks of disease, and the individual has little control over participation in them once they have been implemented.

The target of virtually all these programs is the prevention of disease or injury, a most important objective. They are also an effort to reduce demand for medical services by trying to limit the causes of various diseases. Reduction of demand is one of the better methods of cost containment. However, by limiting attempts at cost containment only to the prevention of disease or injury, these programs barely skim the surface. Even if these programs were completely successful, which they are not, they would not affect the largest amount of disability, which is that induced by psychosocial causes. These account for up to 70 percent of the problems seen daily in physicians' offices.

The direct cost of diagnostic studies performed on patients with emotionally induced symptoms will often exceed the cost of diagnosis in patients who actually have diseases that are causing the symptoms. This is because one of the first few tests performed is apt to be decisive in making a diagnosis when a patient's symptoms are caused by disease, whereas more tests are usually performed for a patient whose symptoms are not related to disease. Of great concern from the economic perspective is the chronic disability often sustained by this large group of patients. This disability manifests itself in many ways, varying from chronic tiredness to chronic pain and from a high rate of absenteeism from work to total inability to work.

For this reason, if health maintenance is to reach its maximum potential as a means of improving the health of the nation and of reducing the aggregate cost of health care in the United States, the concept of health maintenance must be extended considerably beyond its popular definition. The present programs of mass public education must be continued and expanded, but it must also be recognized that there is another important form of health maintenance—dealing with chronic disability from all causes—that should occur daily in physicians' offices on a one-to-one basis. For this to happen, however, physicians and the public at large will have to reexamine their expectations of medical care on the basis of a realistic and appropriate definition of health.

One of the reasons why health has not been viewed as a value judgment is that a sort of mythology has developed in the sciences. Nonmembers of scientific professions may be somewhat awed by the horizons science has opened. These horizons reach the public in the form of various technological tools, and the public is not as aware of the subjective elements of all science; that is, the public may think that all scientists deal only in exact measurements and in judgments based on objective data. This is not the case at all.

John Bleibtreu wrote, "Without a mythology, we must deny mystery, and with this denial, we can only live at great cost to ourselves."[1] Bleibtreu was writing about the

[1] John N. Bleibtreu, *The Parable of the Beast,* Collier Books, New York, 1973, pp. x–xi.

biological sciences in general. In the case of medicine, this mythology may have developed because it is one way of coping with the transience of our being. The mythology develops around the technology, and thus indirectly around the physician who is viewed as controlling that technology. So a middle-aged person who has been a heavy smoker for years may return home and say, "There are no spots on my lungs." Or a diabetic may return home and say, "We finally found the correct insulin dosage." The tone of these statements may be very matter-of-fact, but underlying them is the mystery. Definite measurements allowed the speakers to make the statements, measurements made possible by scientific advances, and those measurements obscured the patients' nonspecific fears or generalized bewilderment about their health.

Bleibtreu continued, "It seems to me that we are in the process of creating a mythology out of the raw materials of science in much the same way that the Greeks and Jews created their mythologies out of the raw materials of history. I feel strongly that this is not only a legitimate, but a necessary process."[1] The status achieved by science, particularly the biological sciences, in the last thirty to forty years is probably immeasurable. Yet as the mythology develops around them, and around medical sciences in particular, the trademarks of medicine may assume proportions larger than life. Medical tools and technology are accepted as infallible, as giving exact determinations of patients' health.

In patient care, this has had some repercussions. The technology has become almost mythological, and the physician may be thought of as someone who is only trained in its use. This may be one reason why many doctors consider health simply as the absence of disease; they, too, are relying heavily on medical technology to describe a patient's health. But in relying on the technology so heavily, other problems have arisen. The reality of patient care, for instance, will frequently fall short of expectations; patients may feel that physicians do not adequately explain things to them, or limited resources may lead to economic and social problems.

The attention given to medicine should be focused more on what physicians do. Possibly, mythology should develop around them. This is not to suggest that physicians should become Olympian figures in our society, but that their function, particularly of primary physicians, should be more widely appreciated. Primary physicians do not use only the medical technology at their disposal. They rely much more heavily on the conceptual skills they have developed and can probably help more than half of their patients without using sophisticated forms of technology at all.

The Medical Interview 7

It is no mere idle philosophy to reflect that, properly communicated, *the patient's complaint does more than point the way to the patient's disease. It is the best expression, the best guide to an understanding of the patient's trouble that we can get to help him. In a real sense, it is his disease.*

Richard M. Magraw, *Ferment in Medicine*

Defining health as a value judgment on which the patient and the physician must ultimately agree would shift the focus of patient care from medical technology to the conceptual skills of the physician. The patient would cease to be a passive subject on whom various tests are performed and instead would assume a more active role in the treatment. The physician would have to draw the patient into discussion, probe for the patient's concerns, and explain what the problems are, if any, and what is causing them. The focus would then be on the physician's ability to accumulate data from the patient and use them effectively.

A single statistic reinforces this: only 30 percent of communication is verbal; the other 70 percent is nonverbal and consists of such things as posture changes, color changes, and changes in facial expressions. Physicians rely heavily on information elicited from their patients, and so the quality of communication between the two is extremely important. A physician's inability to obtain the correct information means that the patient's problem will not be diagnosed as rapidly, or perhaps that it will be diagnosed incorrectly. This may happen because the physician is not attending closely to the patient's nonverbal cues or because the physician will not let the patient say what the trouble really is. Many of these problems need not arise if the medical interview is performed properly.

The interview is the most important part of the physician–patient interaction; it is the device through which the physician learns about the patient's problems and concerns. People may not understand why so much emphasis is placed on the interview in this book, because the interview is usually viewed as a simple conversation. I have had patients tell me that they sometimes felt frustrated by their experiences with physicians because "All we did was talk." But the interview is much more than a simple conversation; it is very dynamic, and that dynamism has to be emphasized. Although 75 to 85 percent of the information a physician needs can be obtained from the interview, it must be remembered that patients are frequently under stress when the interview takes place, possibly affecting the accuracy of the information they give.

Despite its obvious importance, the medical interview has been largely ignored in medical education and research. Only in the last ten years has there been much of an effort to teach medical students how to interview. Interviews performed by medical residents are now sometimes videotaped (with the permission of the patient) and later reviewed and discussed with more experienced physicians. This is a good way of teaching interviewing techniques because the interactions that occur during interviews, when played back on videotape, sometimes astound the students.

Looking at themselves and their patients through the objective lens of the camera, the students recognize the meanings they may have missed, the avenues they did not explore, and the potential information they turned off by interrupting the patient. During the interviews the students were participating and did not have the psychological distance of the videotape. The patients' cues and the direction of the students' questions, which they may not have noticed during the interview, become quite apparent when played back on tape. In the discussion with staff doctors, the students can see where they made their mistakes. Previously, physicians learned of these problems in communication only through experience, but now they are beginning to be taught.

A good medical interview is hard work because the physician is doing much more than merely listening. The physician is attending to the patient's total demeanor and facilitating the description of the patient's symptoms, attitudes, and pattern of living. At the same time the physician is interpreting their meaning. This involves obtaining the patient's spontaneous description of symptoms as well as observing other verbal and nonverbal cues.

Throughout the interview, the physician is also constantly making decisions about the direction the interview should take and thinking about what may be causing the problems being described. At the same time, the physician should suppress the desire to interfere with the patient's description and should encourage the patient to continue speaking. The physician wants information, but it must be information that reflects the patient's true feelings.

For example, I once saw a patient whose bile duct was partially obstructed with a stone, and an infection was developing in the duct and going up into the liver. This is a serious problem in any patient, but was particularly serious in this patient because she was elderly and had diabetes. During the interview she said only once that she felt a little pain. I knew that it was part of her view of life to attach little importance to pain or disability because she was sustained by a great religious faith. Since we did not yet have a diagnosis and surgical exploration of her abdomen was the issue, I felt that it was important to know the intensity of the pain she was experiencing. When I asked her, she said she was unable to describe it; so I asked her if it was just an awareness, an annoyance, or a severe pain. She said that the pain was an annoyance, which could mean that it was no more significant than a bump on the shin. Since a patient's background and attitudes can have a great effect on tolerance of pain, I asked her if there was anything in her life to which she could compare this "annoyance." She said, "It is more annoying than the births of my children were." That statement, more than anything else up to that time, was instrumental in my decision to proceed with the examination, which led to an extensive, but fortunately successful, operation.

The medical interview usually begins with a simple and general question, such as "What can I do for you?" The patient usually responds with a specific complaint, such as "I have a pain in my stomach." This is called the chief complaint, the one that brings the patient to the physician. It may be the patient's chief priority to have that problem resolved, but not always. Sometimes the chief complaint may simply be the "ticket" to get the patient into the sick role and legitimate the visit to the doctor. A patient may, for example, complain to a physician of a pain in the groin or burning while urinating when his real question relates to his concern about impotence. Many patients are reticent about stating their true concerns to physicians, because they fear that they have a disease that could lead to disability or death.

Because the chief complaint may not always reflect the question that caused the patient to consult the physician, the interview should be kept as open as possible. The physician should respond to the patient's first remarks with a statement such as "Tell me about it." This generally initiates the recitation of symptoms, and this recitation should be allowed to proceed with a minimum of interruptions. If it is a truly spontaneous recitation, it will be a description of what the patient is experiencing in the order of importance to the patient. The physician should also try to learn how the patient feels about the situation. The patient will usually mention all these things spontaneously if given the chance. For this to happen, however, the physician must not interrupt, except when necessary to keep the recitation focused on matters of importance to the patient's health.

Examples of open- and closed-style interviews follow:

Open-Style Interview

Physician: What can I do for you?

Patient: I noticed recently that I get chest pain from time to time.

Physician: Tell me about it.

Patient: What do you want to know?

Physician: Whatever you think is important.

Patient: Well, I ran out of gas several weeks ago and had to walk to the filling station. By the time I got there I was feeling a heaviness in the middle of my chest which I never experienced before. Since then, I have gone out each day and walked, and I always get it after a couple of blocks. It makes me stop walking, and when I stop, it goes away fairly quickly. I'm kind of worried about it because my older brother died of a heart attack several years ago. It's different from my brother's pain, however. His pain came at night when he was in bed and he died suddenly two days later. I only get it when I walk or climb a couple flights of stairs. What do you think it is, doctor?

Closed-Style Interview

Physician: What can I do for you?
Patient: I noticed recently that I get chest pain from time to time.
Physician: When did it start?
Patient: Several weeks ago.
Physician: Did you ever have it before that?
Patient: No.
Physician: Is it sharp or dull?
Patient: Well . . .
Physician: Are you short of breath?
Patient: No.
Physician: Is it in the center of your chest? Here? (pointing)
Patient: Yes.
Physician: Does it come with walking?
Patient: Yes.
Physician: How far?
Patient: Two blocks.

Most educators advocate the open style of interviewing. In the examples of interviewing styles just cited, both physicians have learned that the patient has a form of heart disease. The doctor using the open style, however, has obtained additional information about the patient's concern over sudden death. If this concern is not dealt with effectively, the patient may continue to have disabling symptoms despite successful management of the heart disease. Obviously, the concern can not be dealt with until it is recognized.

The open style of interviewing is also preferable if one accepts the view of health as a value judgment, because an open style facilitates the stating of the patients' judgments about their health. This is important to physicians because once patients have made this judgment, they have developed their own priorities for treatment.

It is essential that the physician know what these priorities are in order to obtain the patients' cooperation with treatment. In the example above, the closed style of interviewing does not provide maximum information because it does not reveal the patient's priorities. The patient and the physician bring their own priorities to the interaction based on their definitions of health.

The relationship between the physician's and the patient's priorities is one of the least understood influences on the effectiveness of the medical encounter. A patient may seek a physician for advice about maintaining health, but most patients also have fears, concerns, or questions they expect the physician to address. In other words, they expect certain actions from the physician, and these expectations are always related to their priorities for treatment. As physicians interview and examine their patients, they, too, develop priorities of treatment. Frequently, these priorities are not the same.

Since physicians think that their judgment of the patients' health should prevail, they may assume they do not need to explain to patients why they have developed a specific order of priorities. This is an erroneous assumption. It is essential that they tell their patients when there is a disagreement. Their own priorities must then be justified to the patient. If this is not done, it is usually because the physician either has not taken the time to ascertain the patient's expectations and priorities or is unaware of the importance of recognizing them.

Patients may then cease to feel a part of the interaction. They leave the physician's office feeling as though the physician's advice may be misguided. Their questions have not been answered, their judgment about their health has not been acknowledged, and their priorities have not been recognized. Possibly, if the interview was conducted in a closed style, they may feel somewhat hostile because they were not given the opportunity to express their actual concerns. Studies of the compliance of patients with the recommendations of physicians have shown that patients frequently do not cooperate after they leave the physician's office.[1,2] In some cases half of the prescriptions written were not filled, and half of those filled were not taken according to directions.

Suppose, for example, a patient consults a physician for symptoms caused by an upper respiratory infection at a time when the patient feels that missing work will threaten his or her job security. During the examination, the physician discovers that the patient has moderately high blood pressure which usually requires lifelong treatment to control. The physician knows that the blood pressure problem must be treated, but patients frequently do not agree with this priority because high blood pressure, in its early stages, has no symptoms. In this example, it will be even more difficult to deal with the high blood pressure because the patient's priority is to have the respiratory problem treated so that the job will not be endangered. Therefore, the physician really has three tasks: to deal with the respiratory infection, to formulate a treatment plan for the high blood pressure, and to have the patient cooperate with the recommendations for treating the blood pressure. The physician should first deal with the patient's primary concern—getting back to work—to the patient's satisfaction. It will then be easier to discuss why the treatment of high

[1] R. F. Gillum and A. J. Barsky, "Diagnosis and Management of Patient Noncompliance," *Journal of the American Medical Association*, June 17, 1974, vol. 228, pp. 1563–1567.

[2] Gerry V. Stimson, "Obeying Doctor's Orders: A View from the Other Side," *Social Science and Medicine*, 1974, vol. 8, pp. 97–104.

blood pressure has a high priority, and the patient will be more likely to cooperate with long-term treatment.

One of the reasons medical interviews have not been as effective as they could be is that most physicians practicing medicine today were taught to "pursue symptoms" in an interview. What this term suggests is an adversary setting, similar to a cross-examination in a courtroom, where testimony is distorted by the type of questions asked. What the physician is trying to do in conducting this type of interview is to pursue a specific symptom to a specific organic cause. The Cartesian approach to problem solving requires this type of interview because of its emphasis on reducing things to a simpler level. A problem must have a cause, and that cause will be found when things are reduced to manageable levels. But the goals of a cross-examination in a courtroom are different from the goals of a medical interview, and so it should be apparent that an adversary approach to interviewing has no place in a medical office. Most patients who seek a physician's counsel want to tell what is troubling them. If given the chance, they will describe their problems accurately; it is not necessary or desirable to pursue symptoms. More importantly, patients will describe their problems in their own order of priority.

When a physician pursues symptoms in a closed-style interview, patients usually infer that the physician does not have enough confidence in them to allow them to describe their symptoms in their own words. Under these circumstances, patients may begin to answer questions on the basis of their perceptions of the physician's priorities. This reduces the accuracy of the historical data provided by the patients. It must never be forgotten that patients are the only ones who know what they are experiencing, and it should be left up to them to talk about it in their own words. The physician is there to facilitate the description and to interpret its meaning, but not to influence its content.

When a patient first contacts a physician, two things happen. First, an implicit contract is formed between the two.[3] This contract generally consists of little more than the patient asking the physician for help, and the physician agreeing to try to help. Once this occurs, the physician is committed to the care of that patient unless the physician can find a satisfactory substitute and obtain the patient's agreement to accept the other physician's services. This is an implicit contract, but it is extremely binding. Failure to honor it can place the physician at risk of being sued for abandonment of the patient.

The second thing that happens is that the patient quickly infers what the physician expects. This will color the future relationship between them. It will determine how the patient answers the physician's questions. The patient makes this inference mostly from the kinds of questions the physician asks and from the physician's willingness to listen. In the examples of the two interviewing styles, the patient in the closed interview could conclude that the doctor was interested in the pain pattern but not in other concerns. The doctor may never learn of the patient's fear of dying while asleep.

Most patients perceive these expectations quite accurately. The problem arises when they conform to these expectations, which happens quite easily when patients are under stress. And it is not unusual for patients to feel stress when visiting a physician because of their concerns about their health. The patients may perceive that the physician is not interested in their own description of the problem and would rather expedite the interview by asking questions that are directed toward the physician's preliminary

[3] Richard M. Magraw, *Ferment in Medicine,* W. B. Saunders Co., Philadelphia, 1966, pp. 28–36.

diagnosis. They may then conform to these perceptions by providing what they think the physician wants.

Much has been written about self-fulfilling prophecies, and so it should not be surprising that they can occur in a medical office. Patients feel some stress and are willing to become dependent on the physician if that will resolve their concerns. Under these conditions, patients can be manipulated quite easily, and frequently are. Yet, neither the physician nor the patient may realize that this is happening. In a closed style of interviewing, the physician's diagnostic expectations are controlling the interview, and the patient might easily conform to them. When this happens, the accuracy of the information will suffer. This is analogous to the problem with computers when the input contains mistakes; that is, garbage in, garbage out. Closed questions should be asked only at the end of the interview to clarify details that are medically and behaviorally important, but that the patient may have omitted from the original description.

Information is the most important tool the physician has, and it should be possible to get most of this information from the patient's description of the problem. A well-done interview can eliminate the necessity for many tests that might be performed if adequate historical data are not obtained. Turning patient care into a technological exercise can result in incomplete or erroneous diagnoses, with repetitious testing as well as a lesser degree of patient compliance.

The medical interview is a total interaction between the physician and the patient; it is not limited to a verbal exchange. If physicians are not aware of how their actions can affect the interview, the information they obtain may not be accurate. It is important that the dynamic quality of the interview be understood, because it has been suggested that computers or less well trained personnel perform the medical interview. There is no doubt that a computer could elicit symptoms characteristic of a variety of diseases, but the importance of the interview is that it can, when carried out properly, elicit information about the total patient—responses to symptoms, concerns, how the concerns affect the patient's life, and so on. The interview should be more than an opportunity to pursue symptoms; the physician should also be attending to the total demeanor of the patient as well as listening to the description of the symptoms, and should be trying to learn what the patient's value judgment of his or her health is and what the patient's priorities for treatment are. The physician is preparing to explain to the patient whether those views seem reasonable. Only then is the physician in a position to begin formulating a diagnostic plan.

A computer cannot elicit these types of data. While physician substitutes may be able to do this, they would probably have difficulty interpreting the significance of the data in the clinical setting. Those who suggest the use of computers or less well trained people to perform the interview do not consider the interview to be anything more than a pursuit of symptoms. They do not see it as the dynamic tool that it is. Yet without the interview, the inevitable outcome is excessive reliance on testing and technology with an attendant increase in risk and monetary cost.

The Physician's Tools ______ 8

Nevertheless, both the acquisition and the evaluation of the data can be done with scientific reasoning. Clinicians have complacently accepted the traditional but unproved doctrine that their clinical activities are too human and too complex for science.

Alvan R. Feinstein, *Clinical Judgment*

Once the medical interview is completed, the equally difficult task remains of clarifying the cause of the patient's disorder. This is not simply a problem of choosing the right tests or instruments to make a diagnosis. Blood pressure cuffs, percussion hammers, needles, syringes, scalpels, lighted instruments for looking into various body orifices, and other instruments are at the physician's disposal, but these are really the "givens" of the medical profession. They are aids, but by themselves they do not provide the physician with the answers.

Actually, there are three things that physicians must have at their disposal if they are to be competent: data, knowledge of probabilities, and knowledge of decision logic. If physicians obtain the correct data from the medical interview and subsequent laboratory tests and also understand the significance of those data—which they learn from studying probabilities—they are in a much better position to interpret the data and reach a rational decision about diagnosis and treatment.

The physician is more than an artisan who only needs

to select the proper item from a tool chest to complete a job. Occasionally one suspects that this is how the physician is seen by the public, particularly since only the technological advances of medicine attract most people's attention. The physician who uses this hardware is in the public eye, while the physician who engages in the more deliberate aspects of patient care is relatively unappreciated.

Is the physician a "doer," a user of technology? John Millis addresses himself to this question:

> This is to say that skill is the ultimate aim, but that knowledge is demonstrably relevant to this skill and that the service of the physician is differentiated from that of other professionals, both by what he *does* and also by what he *knows*.
>
> I do not believe that this gap should be attributed to any fundamental failure within medical education. Rather, I believe that the presuppositions which have underlain medical education for a half-century have been made invalid by significant changes in the intellectual world. . . . It would seem that the definition of a professional as a "knowledgeable doer" is only the half-way point in the evolution from a craft to a truly "learned profession." The end point, in my view, is more of a hybrid; one who is both a knower *and* a doer; one in whom the translation of "knowing" into "doing" is personal, creative, and constant; one who lives in both the world of science and of art simultaneously.[1]

Millis' outlook is most interesting. To accept it would mean that the physician would have to be viewed as someone who is as creative as skillful, as knowledgeable as active, and as artistic as scientific. And that is what the primary physician should be. This is because of the three

[1] John S. Millis, *A Rational Public Policy for Medical Education and Its Financing*, National Fund for Medical Education, Cleveland, Ohio, 1977, pp. 47-56.

main tools the primary physician uses: data, knowledge of probabilities, and knowledge of decision logic. Without these, the physician is only a "doer," one who knows more about the hardware than the patient. With them, medicine can become more of a "learned profession."

Let us look at the data the physician requires first. Here, we are defining data quite rigidly into two types. Dr. Richard Magraw classified these types as primary and secondary. The primary data are defined as the information obtained from the patient, including data acquired from the medical interview, data acquired during the physical examination, and data from laboratory tests of all types.

Secondary data are the things that are part of the physician's background. This includes medical education, certainly, but also all those things that are learned experientially, from reading, from attending conferences, and from discussions with colleagues. These data form the framework with which the primary data will be compared.

Medical education emphasizes the secondary data, and possibly most people would think of this as proper. Physicians, and the public as well, realize the hazards of inaccurate secondary data. But what if the primary data are wrong? What if the medical interview did not provide accurate information or was misinterpreted by the physician? Inaccurate primary data will always lead to an incorrect diagnosis, regardless of how complete the secondary data are. It is appalling to me that people are not aware of the hazards of inaccurate primary data, but this lack of awareness is understandable for the following reasons:

1. The medical interview, which accounts for 70 to 85 percent of the primary data, is *entirely subjective*. In addition, it is held at a time of considerable emotional stress for the patient. Frequently, the greater the patient's perception of the problem, the greater is the stress to the patient.

More significantly perhaps, the patient has adopted the sick role and is thus willingly dependent on the physician. This dependence will sometimes alter the accuracy of the history, as we saw in the preceding chapter, because the patient's description of symptoms can be influenced by the physician's demeanor. In this situation, patients will sometimes subconsciously try to please their physician by giving the answers they think the physician will like.

Adding to the subjectivity of the interview, the physician's interpretation of the patient's description may also be influenced by whatever educational or cultural differences may exist between the physician and the patient.

2. Primary data obtained from the physical examination are considerably more objective than those acquired from the interview. But even here a certain amount of subjective data will be gathered. The best examples of these are the patient's responses to painful or other sensory stimuli. Here again, the interpretation of these data is influenced by the physician's knowledge of psychology and sociology.

3. Laboratory data are usually viewed as being totally objective, but they also have to be interpreted for their probable significance to a specific patient. The physician must first consider the possibility of human error when a test result is received. While this can be kept to a minimum, there will always be an irreducible amount of human error in even the best of laboratories.

A second problem in interpreting laboratory data is a little less obvious. This is related to the definition of the "normal" and "abnormal" values of a particular test. It occasionally becomes a problem because a normal test result and an abnormal test result are determined arbitrarily in biological testing. What this means is that a patient who is not ill may occasionally have an abnormal test, and a patient who is diseased may have a normal test. This is quite important, because it means that even after the physician accepts the technical accuracy of a test, it is necessary to decide whether the result is significant to the patient's particular problem. The physician has to consider the probability of whether the test accurately indicates the presence or absence of disease by determining the position of the test result on the normal (Gaussian) curve and then by relating this to the patient's description of the problem.

This is why the medical interview is so important. Physicians must elicit accurate information during the interview if subsequent laboratory tests are to be interpreted accurately. The process of diagnosing is a sequential one (Fig. 1). Physicians apply the primary data obtained from the interview in the interpretation of certain data from the physical examination. They then use primary data from both the interview and the physical examination to select laboratory tests, and use the accumulated primary data to determine whether enough studies have been performed to make decisions about treatment or whether more data and studies are required. They may also decide that they should acquire more secondary data by such means as library research or consultation.

Throughout this sequence, physicians must keep in mind that laboratory data are statistical data and must be interpreted as such; that is, the significance of a specific test result will vary from patient to patient. Physicians must take this variability and its causes into account if they are to be of maximum help to the patient.

There are three concepts of which physicians must be aware if they are to interpret the laboratory data accurately: the normal range of a test, the sensitivity and specificity of a test, and the predictive value of a test. Laboratory data are not as objective as most people think, and the following will explain why.

Consider the normal range of values first. In biological testing, when test results are called normal, it usually means

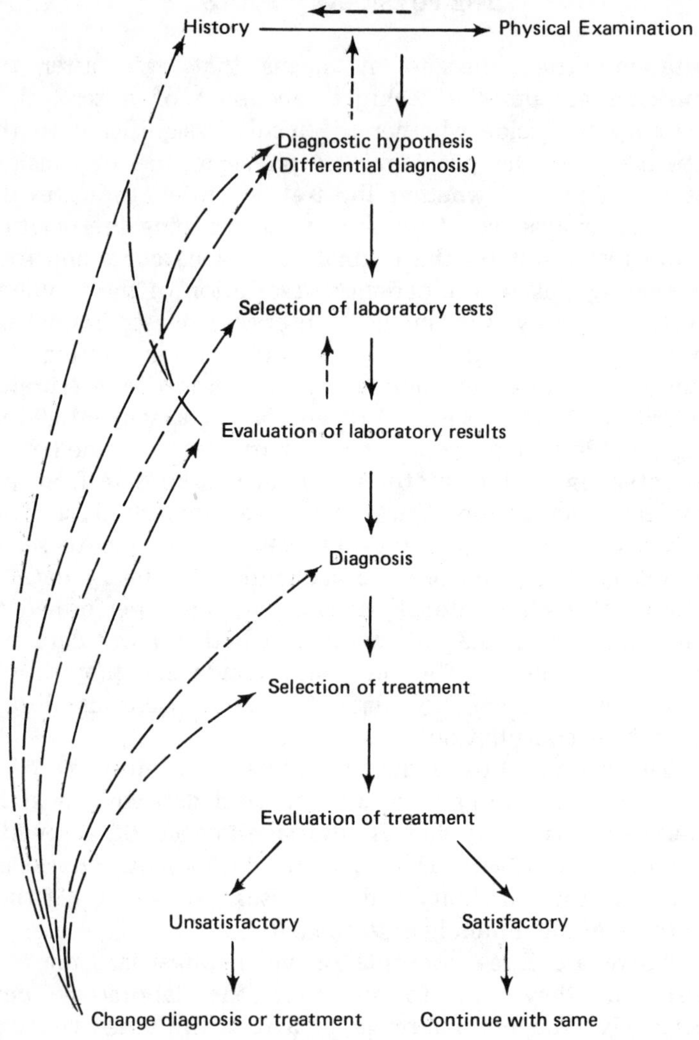

Figure 1 Any deficiency in acquiring primary data, interpreting them, synthesizing them with secondary data, or estimating probabilities can result in erroneous diagnoses or ineffective treatment. The process must then be repeated with overutilization of time, testing, medication, and so on.

that the specific disease being tested for is not present. However, not all test results in normal people (people who do not have the disease) fall into a sharply defined category separate from the test results of abnormal people (people who have the disease being tested for). At both ends of the range of possible values for a test (high and low values), there is an inevitable blending of the test results of those who have the disease and those who do not. In other words, the test result ceases to be decisive at both extremes of the range.

To help resolve this problem, the normal range of a test came to be defined by its position on the normal curve. An arbitrary decision was made to define the normal range of a biological test by placing the upper and lower limits of a normal test result two standard devisions from the mean. Basically, what it means is that in a healthy population being tested for a certain disease, 95 percent would fall within the normal range and 5 percent would fall outside it. These 5 percent would be at risk of being considered to have the disease if the test result were the only criterion used to make the diagnosis.

The concept of a normal range of values for biological tests is a good one. With it, the test results can be compared with the data elicited during the medical interview and the physical examination. Even when a patient's test is normal, but falls near the outer limits of the normal range, it frequently brings the physician closer to the diagnosis. This is particularly true when the diagnosis is also suggested by other data from the history and the physical examination. It is important, however, to remember that the method used to define normal ranges means that $2\frac{1}{2}$ percent of the people who do not have the disease will fall outside the normal upper limits for the test and $2\frac{1}{2}$ percent of the people who do not have the disease will fall below the lower limits for the test. In other words, 5 percent of the people who do not have the disease will have abnormal results. These are called false positive results and frequently require further testing if the condition of the patient is to be accurately determined.

Another way of looking at this is through the concept of sensitivity and specificity of tests. The sensitivity of a test is defined as the percentage of patients who have the disease and who have a positive test result. If 100 people with a certain disease are tested with a test that has a sensitivity of 0.95, then 95 of those people will have a positive result and 5 will have a negative result. These five have false negative results, and there is a risk that these patients may be untreated unless someone does not believe the test on the basis of other data.

Specificity of a test is defined as the percentage of people who do not have the disease who will have a negative result. For example, if a test for a certain disease has a specificity of 0.85, and if 100 patients who do not have the disease are given the test, 85 of them will have a negative result and 15 will have a positive result. These 15 have false positive test results, and the only alternatives available for these patients are either to be treated for the disease when they actually do not have it, or to undergo further tests to disprove the initial tests.

The sensitivity and specificity of a particular test are also determined arbitrarily, but there is one important principle concerning their relationship to each other that must be clearly understood: they are inversely related. As the specificity of a test decreases, its sensitivity increases, and vice versa. In other words, reducing the risk of false positives increases the risk of false negatives, and reducing the risks of false negatives increases the risk of false positives.

Physicians who understand this inverse relationship can utilize it so that a test will have maximum usefulness in clinical medicine. Suppose, for example, that a test is done for a disease that is extremely dangerous and that the treatment of the disease is simple and safe. A deliberate choice can be made to increase the sensitivity of the test, which will result in fewer false negative results. This is done simply by redefining what results will be abnormal. More people who have the disease will then have test results that show them to have the disease. But since sensitivity and specificity are inversely related, there will also be a larger number of false positive test results—some people who do not have the disease will have results that show them to have it. These patients will also receive treatment unless the diagnosis of the illness is disproved by further testing or by other data that the physician has collected. Acute appendicitis is a disease where such a deliberate choice has been made. It is considered acceptable to overdiagnose acute appendicitis to the extent that 10 to 15 percent of appendectomies are performed on people who have normal appendices but have abdominal pain from some other cause. This is acceptable because the risk of a ruptured appendix far exceeds the risk of the surgical procedure.

On the other hand, there are some diseases for which the risks or discomfort of treatment in the early stages preclude treating patients with false positive results. For these diseases, especially if it is not important whether the disease is treated before or after its presence becomes apparent, the sensitivity and specificity of the test will be defined in such a way that there will be fewer false positive results and more false negatives.

These manipulations only form the base of a doctor's statistical knowledge. In fact, if knowledge of the specificity, sensitivity, and normal range of a test were all that was necessary to interpret test results, it would be a relatively straightforward exercise. This is particularly true since the limits defining them can be established arbitrarily. These are not the only variables, however. The last variable, the predictive value, if not clearly understood, really throws a monkey wrench into the works.

Probably the most important statistical variable in clinical medicine is the predictive value of a test. This is defined as the percentage of people who have a positive test result and who also have the disease. It defines the reliability of the test in a clinical setting.

The predictive value of a test is determined by three variables: the sensitivity of the test, its specificity, and the prevalence of the disease in the patient population being tested. The sensitivity and specificity of a test are determined arbitrarily before the test is given. The question now is how to manipulate the nature of the patient population in order to maintain a high predictive value for a specific test. It can be done, and it can be shown that the predictive value of a test will increase as the prevalence of the disease being tested for in that population increases.[2]

Consider, for example, a test for a disease in a population in which 50 percent of the people have the disease. Using a test with a sensitivity and a specificity of 0.95, the predictive value of that test would be 95 percent (see Table 1). This means that 95 of 100 people being tested who had a positive result would prove to have the disease and only 5 of 100 people who had a positive result would have false positives. This is a very reliable test.

Now consider the same test given to a population in which only 1 percent of the people have the disease. In this population, the predictive value of the test would be only 16 percent! Of every 100 people in this population who had a positive result, only 16 would have the disease, while 84 would be healthy. This is critically important, not only because it is possible to avoid these situations, but also because their occurrence means that the patients with false positive results have to either undergo more testing, with its attendant risk and discomfort, or be treated for a disease they do not have.

[2] This is derived from Bayes' theorem.

Table 1 Predictive value of a test with a sensitivity and specificity of 0.95 in a population of 10,000 in which the prevalence of the disease is 1 percent[a]

Number of people	Number of positive results	Number of negative results
100 diseased	95	5
9,900 nondiseased	495	9,405
10,000 total	590	9,410

Results: 95 positive
495 false positive
Predictive value = 95/590
= 16 percent

[a]Change prevalence to 10 percent and predictive value = 68 percent. Change prevalence to 50 percent and predictive value = 95 percent.

This is why conceptually oriented physicians have to live in the world of predictive value. Knowledge of these sorts of probabilities enables them to better handle the data elicited. Every patient they see brings them a new challenge, for not only do they have to obtain about three-quarters of their data from a subjective source, but they have to be able to develop an individual plan for each patient by using the data properly.

These statistics may be difficult to understand. The purpose of this chapter is not to impress people with the quantitative problems that physicians face every day. Instead, people should understand that physicians frequently have to make decisions that are not based on rigid data. If that were not the case, patient care would be much less of a challenge.

The secondary data physicians learn are also necessary and important. However, it is equally important for the public to realize that few tests have been devised that will tell a physician with absolute certainty that a patient has a particular disease. Most diagnoses result instead from a synthesis of various kinds of data. The synthesis, in turn, is dependent on the individual physician's knowledge of all of the conceptual skills that make up what used to be called the "art of medicine." Each patient is unique and brings an individual constellation of signals to the physician. The physician must discover a pattern in these signals and use it to formulate a proper plan of treatment.

As Millis said, skill is the ultimate aim. But more importantly, the physician must know when to use that skill and also know which skill to use. With the great technology available, we may all think that the physician only needs to use that technology to do the job properly. However, if the intellectual tools can be mastered, the technological tools will be used less frequently. They will also be used more appropriately. The number of unnecessary laboratory tests will be reduced; therapeutic procedures will be used less often as physicians come to rely more on their conceptual skills.

Since no one really wants to rely on a test with a predictive value of only 16 percent, it is important that physicians be taught that they are able to concentrate the prevalence of any disease in the population they are testing. They can do this by carefully collecting their primary data, by accumulating a solid base of secondary data, and by judiciously synthesizing the two.

The Physician's Commodity 9

At such a time [in the face of differences of opinion by important advisors], he can do no more than to retire "into his tent" and assess the bases of decision. He has finished with advice.

Walter Bedell Smith, *Eisenhower's Six Great Decisions*

The preceding chapter should dispel the notion that physicians work against great odds. Quite the opposite is true; physicians who understand probabilities can work quite closely with the odds and reduce long shots to better-than-even chances. They can interpret their data in such a way that the raw numbers will have more significance for individual patients. This is one of the most important things physicians do, one of the things that could define their function. But it is not understood as well as other, more conspicuous activities in which physicians engage, partly because it is not as awe-inspiring as some forms of medical technology and partly because medical education has not focused on this aspect of patient care as intensely as it has on the use of medical technology.

What has developed is an image of physicians as technologists, of physicians who engage in various discrete activities in diagnosing and treating patients; that is, a particular physician might check one's vision, or give physical examinations and advice, or prescribe drugs, or perform surgery. When people think of physicians, it is usually in terms of what they do. But if someone were to ask you what primary physicians do, it would be very difficult to define their function in such specific terms. That is because they are physicians who are mainly selling decisions. They use a variety of technological tools, and they also send their patients, when necessary, to physicians in more limited specialties. But those tools and referrals are really incidental to their function. Their main tools are data and probabilities, and their main commodity is decisions.

Decisions are made throughout the course of performing the history and physical examination. Decisions are made about the kind and number of diagnostic studies necessary, and about whether consulting other specialists is necessary. Decisions are made about the nature of the treatment to be prescribed and, of course, about the extent of that treatment.

In the simplest terms, these decisions focus on whether a patient is suffering from a nonthreatening, self-limited disease that requires only brief treatment, from a serious illness that can be treated and cured, or from an untreatable, rapidly progressive, fatal disease. Most patients will fall between the extremes on this continuum and will only raise the question of which diagnostic and therapeutic procedures would be most effective. But for these patients, as well as for the patients at the extremes, whatever decisions the physician makes will determine the extent of diagnostic and therapeutic procedures and thus the cost to that patient.

The extent of treatment patients receive should be determined by the primary physician. Therefore, primary physicians who can make sound decisions are urgently needed. The monetary costs of unnecessary diagnostic tests and unnecessary therapeutic regimens do add up, whether it is over an individual patient's lifetime or whether it is the aggregate cost to society. The problem has developed to its present state because in the last three decades medical science has increased the knowledge of disease processes so much that practicing physicians now have a wide number of choices available for any problems patients bring to them. As recently as the 1930s, for instance, electrocardiography and X-ray were in their infancy; sulfa drugs had just been discovered to be useful (there were no other effective forms of specific, anti-infectious chemotherapy available); and pneumococcal pneumonia was still being treated largely with serum and had a high mortality rate. So when pre-World War II physicians were faced with patients who were critically ill, they would probably use all the resources at their disposal in order to try to intervene successfully.

Their alternatives, however, were quite limited, while modern physicians have a multitude of alternatives. They should not use all the resources at their disposal because it would subject patients to too much suffering as well as exorbitant costs. Yet, like the physicians of the 1930s, modern physicians do want to do whatever they can; like their predecessors, they frequently still like to say, "Everything has been done that *can* be done."

The artistic and creative physician described by John Millis is needed to help change this emphasis on using all, or even most of, the available resources. Physicians should be saying, "Everything has been done that *should* be done." Fortunately, physicians—although many times only at the individual patient's request—are moving in this direction.

If the current trend toward diagnostic and therapeutic excess is to be reversed, however, more physicians of a different type are needed than are being educated today. These physicians will have to be intellectuals, dealing largely with intellectual tools; they will have to have well-developed conceptual skills; and they will have to have the confidence and courage necessary to follow their decisions through, even when faced with difficult dilemmas.

It is a question of judgment, and physicians should be able to say that no more should be done when such a decision is in the best interest of the patient.

Thoughtful physicians will do this. They will be able to decide not to follow a course of action and deal with the greater emotional strain that this decision entails. This will put to the test their patience, courage, and self-restraint, as well as those of the patient and the patient's family. Humans are still mortal, and there will come a time in everyone's life when medicine and physicians can do no more. At that point, someone should say "Stop!"

Not all of a physician's decisions will deal with terminal illness. We have already seen how a physician may decide during the course of an interview that a patient's problems are psychologically caused. And we saw in Chapter 1 that it may be wiser for a physician to take a drastic course of action than to try to do all that might be possible. Today, physicians confront more and more problems because their technology enables them to do something. But the question of whether something *should* be done remains unanswered.

That is really the challenge confronting American medicine today. Some physicians have to be in firm control of the technology and be in a position to decide that no more should be done. This is not the case today, because the physicians with the highest status—the ones the public hears about, the ones most medical students learn from—are those whose function is largely defined by the technology of their specialty. The public is much more familiar, for example, with heart transplantation than with the dynamics of medical decision making. What is needed is to develop a physician model—the primary physician—and allow that physician to make the decisions about the treatment for each patient.

This could be very difficult to achieve, not only because of the way medical students and residents have been taught, but also because of the difficulties of deciding *not* to pursue treatment further. This is where decision making becomes crucial. Perhaps it would be helpful to look fairly closely at the dynamics of making a medical decision.

I prefer to define decisions quite narrowly, as choices between two alternatives. A physician may be working with several hypotheses in any situation, but there are only two choices for each hypothesis: the physician can accept any particular hypothesis or reject it. For each patient whose symptoms may indicate a number of diseases, the physician must establish the hypotheses and then proceed to accept or reject each one.

Thus, there are only two kinds of errors a physician can make: rejecting the hypothesis when it should have been accepted (alpha error), or accepting the hypothesis when it should have been rejected (beta error). Another way of describing these two types of errors is to call them errors of commission and errors of omission. The physicians who treated the woman mentioned in Chapter 1 made an error of commission; they tried to restore the circulation in one leg when this should not have been attempted. Most physicians' errors are of this type, as we shall see.

Statisticians say that a decision maker who is correct more than 50 percent of the time is good at making decisions. Physicians, however, are uncomfortable with that statement for obvious reasons. One could, since decisions are choices between two alternatives, guess which alternative to choose and, with luck, be right 50 percent of the time. Therefore, physicians collect various data to try to improve their chances of making correct decisions, but the data are mostly subjective and easily misinterpreted. The data will help in making decisions, but to do so they must be interpreted; and to interpret them, they must be placed in the appropriate context. The medical interview, for example, is the richest source of data, but these data have to be interpreted carefully if they are to have any useful meaning. Whether they are correctly interpreted is subject to many variables, even assuming the patient's ability to describe symptoms accurately and the physician's ability to understand the patterns of that patient's life.

Beyond the medical history, the data physicians accumulate also tend to be subjective and interpretative. Laboratory data, as we saw in the preceding chapter, do not always have the credibility that people generally think they have. They are not accepted for what they say, but instead are interpreted within a framework that the physician has established. In fact, data that may be accurate and significant one day may be less relevant the next day should the situation change at all overnight.

These reasons help explain why it is difficult to make medical decisions. But the most obvious reason has not really been discussed, and it may very well be the most important one: the physician is making decisions about a human being, decisions that may affect that person and his or her family. The pressures that physicians experience as a result may be one of the major causes of poor decision making.

What physicians frequently do, because of the possibility of errors in their interpretation of the medical interview and laboratory data and because of the pressure they feel, is deliberately select the type of error that will occur. When they do this, they almost invariably select the error of commission; that is, they choose an extra diagnostic procedure or an extra treatment rather than choose to do nothing. They want to do everything that can be done.

Uncritical decisions of this sort, however, do not take into account all the data that have been collected, and thus a major part of the decision-making process is faulty. There is no way a physician can completely eliminate the possibility of errors in the interpretation of primary data, but the physician should not try to correct the interpretation by consistently selecting the error of commission. In fact, consistent selection of one type of error increases the total error.

Instead, a good decision maker, while recognizing that the evaluation of the primary data may be wrong, will select an acceptable limit of total error with only a highly selective regard for the type of error that may be made. The acceptable limit of total error will vary from one disease to another and also from one patient to another, even if the patients have the same disease. The limit is determined after careful consideration of the natural history of the patient's disease, the general condition of the patient, and the risks and benefits of the contemplated tests or treatment. In other words, it is based on the physician's estimate of the risks and benefits of the various alternatives. Only after considering these things should one look at the type of error that may be involved.

The situation of each patient needs to be assessed individually; the total disease pattern needs to be known. The course of treatment for the woman mentioned in Chapter 1 was not based on this. There was a remote possibility that reconstructive surgery could help the leg, but the total risk to her far exceeded the possible benefit. This was known before the decision to try to reconstruct her circulation was made; yet the physicians chose to make an error of commission—they chose to perform this procedure. The acceptable limit of error for her situation was really quite low if they had chosen to amputate both legs immediately. They might have been wrong, but if they had been, her general condition would not have changed. She would still have been confined to a wheelchair.

Errors of commission always increase the monetary cost and frequently the risk to the patient. This has become a major cause of iatrogenic (physician-induced) illnesses. Different forces combine to cause physicians to choose the error of commission when they make their final decisions about treatment or diagnostic tests. Even the threat of malpractice suits and the third party guarantor are partially responsible. In one case, physicians may be practicing a defensive sort of medicine. In the other case, they may think that, since an insurance company or the government is paying, the financial burden will be less onerous. But from a societal point of view, that reasoning is specious.

A certain amount of error is inevitable, but the amount can be reduced by selecting an acceptable limit of total error rather than by uncritically selecting a type of possible error. Implicit in this is that in patient care, deliberate and careful choices must be made because of the technological capacity of modern medicine. Physicians must control the use of these tools in all situations, and the essence of that control lies in the ability to make good decisions. Thus, decisions are the primary physician's main commodity.

Dilemmas in Patient Care 10

Is it true that the concepts of science and those of ethics and values belong to different worlds? Is the world of what is *subject to test, and is the world of* what ought to be *subject to no test? I do not believe so.*

J. Bronowski, *Science and Human Values*

It may seem that a heavy burden is placed on primary physicians. They are asked to spend the necessary time to acquire the primary data, to interpret them, and to make decisions based on them. And there will be times when this will lead to a dilemma. All types of physicians confront dilemmas, but primary physicians will be expected to resolve most of these dilemmas satisfactorily—even when that requires examination of the ill-defined area of stopping treatment.

When should physicians stop treating a patient? At what point in the course of a terminal illness is dying irreversible? At what point in the course of a terminal illness can a physician no longer help? Is a patient dead who requires artificial life support systems to maintain autonomic functions and has no chance of regaining consciousness? These are the sorts of questions that are usually thought of as the moral questions physicians must answer. Anytime a physician withholds treatment or stops heroic treatment, it is usually thought that the physician made a moral judgment. Is this true? There is no question that physicians are often caught in a dilemma—that the problem a patient poses has no satisfactory solution. But does this necessarily mean that the decisions that are made are moral or ethical judgments? In caring for a dying patient, must a physician always make a moral judgment before modifying or stopping treatment?

An interesting example of this problem was reported in a recent issue of the *New England Journal of Medicine.*[1] The article described how the staff of the Burn Center at the University of Southern California Medical Center handles burn patients who have no hope of survival. The actions described in the article raised some questions that were widely discussed in daily newspapers and national magazines, and the conclusions reached by the authors were generally praised.

During 1975 and 1976, 748 patients were admitted to the Burn Center, and of those 126 died. The article discussed 24 of the patients who died. These 24 were injured so severely that the physicians knew that they would die. The inevitability of death in these patients was based on very decisive data. The basic requirement for this conclusion was that careful comparison of the condition of these patients with that of patients previously admitted with similar extensive burns revealed that no similarly injured patients had ever survived. In other words, death had to be a certain outcome before a patient was included in this study.

The staff then approached these patients in the following manner:

> In an attempt to establish a relationship with the patient, the attending physician or resident under his guidance tries to

[1] Sharon H. Imbus and Bruce E. Zawacki, "Autonomy for Burned Patients When Survival is Unprecedented," *New England Journal of Medicine,* August 11, 1977, vol. 297, pp. 308–310.

> assume the role of a compassionate friend who is willing to listen. Hands are held, and an effort is made to look deeply into the patient's eyes to perceive the unspoken questions that may lie there. Nonverbal cues are watched for closely.[2]

After establishing this close relationship, the staff informed the patients that survival with injuries like theirs was unprecedented and that they must decide whether they wanted the physicians to try to save them or simply to comfort them during the last hours of life. (Severely burned patients are quite lucid for several hours after being injured and can understand what they are being told.) Twenty-one patients chose to be comforted. Three requested that heroic measures be taken to try to save them. Those three also died.

It is praiseworthy that 21 patients were spared being needlessly subjected to heroic treatment. This represents a major advance in the care of the terminally ill. But what of the other three? There still seems to be an inconsistency here. If it was true that death was inevitable when these patients entered the Burn Center (and the data provided by the authors certainly indicate that it was) what did the physicians have to offer these patients beyond maintenance of comfort and dignity?

Because of the cloudiness surrounding the subject of dilemmas, let us examine this question closely. Dilemmas that occur during the course of medical practice have become a subject of intense public scrutiny and concern. A number of books and many papers have been written on this subject in recent years, and a number of groups have been organized to study various problems in medical ethics. This increased scrutiny and concentrated study are welcome. One can rejoice over the fact that these matters

[2] Reprinted by permission from *New England Journal of Medicine*, vol. 297, p. 308, 1977.

are beginning to be approached more analytically than they have been in the past.

Since decisions have to be made, physicians are inevitably faced with dilemmas. When this happens, there are frequently pressures on the physician to continue treatment even beyond the point where it seems justifiable, and some of these situations attract extensive publicity. Many of these problems grab the popular imagination because they suggest uncontrolled technology. In these instances, the physicians appear to be little more than knowledgeable doers who cannot guide the technology that their science has created. But there is far more to the subject of dilemmas than these situations, important and dramatic as they are.

It is unfortunate that most dilemmas in medical practice are called moral or ethical dilemmas, when in reality they are not. This error has probably come about because dilemmas that occur in patient care have the potential for affecting the future well-being of another person. However, this is not a sufficient reason for classifying a dilemma as a moral or ethical one.

Actually, there are two kinds of dilemmas that occur in patient care—medical dilemmas and moral dilemmas. Since dilemmas are common in medical practice, this distinction is important because the kinds of data necessary to resolve medical dilemmas are quite different from the kinds of data necessary to resolve moral dilemmas.

Medical dilemmas can be resolved decisively by the responsible physician on the basis of careful interpretation and evaluation of all the clinical data that are available. An attempt is made by the physician to use these data to obtain a risk/benefit ratio that is the most advantageous to the patient. The physician makes a decision on this basis and makes recommendations to the patient and/or the patient's family. The patient and the family are strong participants in the interaction in that they make the ultimate choice of accepting the recommendations or rejecting them (by requesting consultation or by changing doctors).

On the other hand, moral dilemmas occur in situations in which a risk/benefit ratio cannot be determined decisively because too many of the risk alternatives and benefit alternatives become value judgments on the part of the decision maker. In other words, in moral dilemmas the clinical data are inconclusive. The available clinical data will not yield an answer to the problem, and the resolution is dependent on a value judgment of some sort; the physician is unable to make a decision solely on the basis of the biomedical data. Certain values, such as the quality and expected duration of life, have to be considered also. These kinds of dilemmas may be very difficult to resolve.

It is imperative that these two kinds of dilemmas be distinguished and dealt with separately if clarity of discussion and clarity of decision making are to be attained, because each calls for a different kind of resolution. Although ethicists are working diligently to develop and teach approaches to the resolution of difficult moral dilemmas, satisfactory methods are not yet available. On the other hand, medical dilemmas can be resolved by knowledgeable physicians as they carefully elicit and analyze the clinical data.

It seems to be widely thought that in very grim situations physicians are always making moral judgments, that they are deciding who will live and who will die. Moral dilemmas are often viewed as dilemmas that are caused by an uncontrolled technology. In the Burn Center, this dilemma was interpreted as a moral one and resolved by allowing the 24 patients to choose whether to be subjected to medical technology. The patients made value judgments in this case.

In my opinion, however, the report from the Burn Center is an example of the tendency to mistake medical dilemmas for moral dilemmas. In the patients presented, the clinical data answered the question decisively. All 24 were going to die. If the attending physicians had viewed each of these problems as a medical dilemma, all 24 would have been spared useless heroic treatment. It was not necessary to invoke value judgments in this situation.

Some will say that patients should participate in making the kind of choices involved in the situation at the Burn Center. I am a firm believer in patient participation and agree that patients should always participate in decisions when difficult choices must be made. In this situation, however, I do not see any choice. It is postulated in the article that death had to be inevitable for the patients to be included in the study. By definition, then, there could be no definitive treatment for any of those patients. Comforting the patients and preserving dignity was the only choice available.

If we remove the argument from a situation with a tragic outcome to more common types of decisions, the point becomes clearer. As an absurd example, imagine a physician saying to a healthy patient on whom he has just completed a comprehensive examination, "I have never seen acute appendicitis in anyone as healthy and free of symptoms as you are, nor have I been able to find any such reports. However, there is a very remote chance that the data are wrong and that your appendix could rupture tonight. Therefore, I am offering you two alternatives. You may go on about the business of living your life and come to me only when you need further medical help or advice. On the other hand, if you do not wish to live with the uncertainty, small as it is, of having a ruptured appendix, I will remove it."

The major difference affecting the decision making for the hypothetical patient as compared to the burn patients is the seeming inevitability of a period of healthy life as compared to the seeming inevitability of death. In the healthy patient, it would not occur to anyone to overrule the medical evidence and suggest treatment that adds to discomfort without adding benefit.

Why should there be this tendency to classify medical dilemmas as moral dilemmas? One can only speculate, but there are perhaps three reasons.

The first reason stems from the ubiquitous fear of error. All physicians know that there are few absolutes in medical practice, and that there will inevitably be errors. A physician faced with a dilemma is haunted by this fear of error. It is very difficult for physicians to make these decisions, just as it is frequently difficult for families to accept them. If a situation calls for drastic and irreversible action (such as loss of a limb or not using life support technology), it is very tempting to discuss value judgments rather than available data. The result may then be that the physician decides not to impose a value judgment on the patient. This, in turn, almost uniformly results in a second decision, which is to do something rather than not do it. Through this circuitous route, errors of commission are selected as the preferred type of error, and thus total error will increase. This not only may be hard on such patients, but also results in increased use of medical resources. The overall quality of care is worsened.

The second reason is that it is difficult to determine when a medical decision becomes a value judgment. Does a 10 percent chance of saving a leg from immediate amputation justify multiple surgical procedures in an elderly woman with crippling arthritis who is confined to a wheelchair? How vigorously should a patient with terminal lung disease be treated when the probable life expectancy, should the patient recover from the acute problem, is about two months of marginal life confined to a bedroom with an oxygen tank. At some point, value judgments enter into the decision. When this happens, the patient and the patient's family must be included in the decision-making process. However, when the family becomes involved in medical decision making beyond simply accepting or rejecting the physician's recommendations, the complexity of the problem increases. This is because these kinds of decisions are usually associated with severe illnesses where death is the probable outcome. Therefore, the physician must attempt to spare the family as much guilt as possible. This can be done only if the physician assumes major responsibility for all the decisions, even while learning of the family's wishes.

A third important reason for the confusion between medical and moral dilemmas may be that we do not like to consider the fact that everyone dies sooner or later, and that most people succumb at the end stage of one form of disease or another. We seem to have forgotten that, at some point, the process of dying becomes acute and irreversible and that a knowledgeable physician is in the best position to recognize when such an irreversible end stage has begun. Because of the effectiveness of artificial life support systems, the end stages of disease can sometimes be extensively prolonged. We must be aware that skilled diagnosticians are usually able to identify irreversibility with a high degree of accuracy, and that it may be ill-advised to initiate life support systems as often as we currently do.

A panel discussion was presented at a recent meeting of the American College of Physicians, entitled "Who Shall Live? Who Decides?" It quickly became apparent that few physicians present cared to be represented as deciding who shall live or not live. The reason for their reluctance is that physicians in their daily practice should make (and usually do make) their decisions on the basis of the available data, even those concerning whether to initiate heroic treatment. These data include the primary data acquired from the patient and the secondary data. Of the secondary data, the most important are those which describe the natural history of the disease (if left untreated) and the effectiveness of each type of available treatment.

Their responsibility is to elicit as much data concerning their patient's condition as is necessary to decide whether further treatment will effect improvement and, if so, what kind of treatment to use. If their decision is that further treatment will not be useful and will only increase the patient's suffering, then they should decide to discontinue all treatment except what will make the patient comfortable. This process in no way implies that physicians decide who shall live or who shall die when they make such a decision.

Unquestionably, there is considerable overlap between medical and moral dilemmas. In reality, the resolutions of most medical dilemmas have moral implications, and the resolutions of most moral dilemmas have medical implications. This overlap is part of the very nature of patient care. Even with agreement on the medical data, conscientious physicians may disagree about a plan of treatment. In spite of the overlap, it is important to keep the two types of dilemmas separate, as this will result in a much larger proportion of dilemmas being recognized as medical rather than moral. It will permit more precise decision making and patient care will benefit.

Cardiopulmonary resuscitation and utilization of various forms of life support systems in intensive care units and coronary care units exemplify the gray area between medical and moral dilemmas that exists in the minds of many people, including physicians. This need not be so. For example, a competent physician can nearly always predict the outcome of a cardiac arrest before initiating cardiac resuscitation and before putting the patient on an artificial life support system, if the physician knows the medical history of the patient. Decisions on whether to initiate extraordinary measures should be made on the basis of the medical data. They should be medical decisions and should not be regarded as moral decisions.

If the distinction between medical and moral dilemmas were more widely recognized—by both physicians and patients—there would probably be a reduction in the overuse of medical technology. There would be an associated reduction in the duration of patient suffering, the mental anguish of the patient's family during this period of extreme illness, and the cost to society.

Organ transplantation is a different kind of example. Kidney transplantation is the most advanced of the various forms of organ transplantation and lends itself to discussion.

When considering kidney transplantation and the problems of decision making associated with it, one has to separate consideration of the recipient of the transplant from consideration of the donor. With regard to the recipient, most of the decisions to be made are medical decisions. Many dilemmas arise in the selection of recipients for kidney transplantation, but these are mostly medical dilemmas. They can be decided on the basis of the responsible physician's knowledge of the probable natural history of the disease in the patient who is ill and whether the patient has any other disease that may be life threatening. These are sometimes difficult decisions, to be sure; that is why they are called dilemmas. But they are not moral dilemmas.

The donor of the kidney presents a different kind of problem. Donors are selected in one of two ways. The living donor is selected from healthy members of the patient's family to donate one kidney. The donor agrees to submit to the immediate risk of an operative procedure plus the long-term risk of living with only one kidney. The long-term risk is uncertain to date. Should the donor develop kidney disease similar to the kidney disease of the recipient (who is closely related to the donor) only half the normal amount of kidney tissue would be present. Also, the risk of entering old age with only one kidney compared to having both kidneys is unknown at the present time. Consequently, selection of a living donor presents a moral dilemma that has to be resolved if the transplant is to occur. At present this decision cannot be made solely on the basis of medical data.

The second kind of donor is a cadaver donor. The use of cadaver donors is one of the main reasons that death has been redefined as brain death. The cadaver donor is usually an otherwise healthy person who has sustained some sudden injury that has led to irreversible brain damage. He is maintained on artificial life support up to the time of the transplant. Then, life support is ended and the kidney is transplanted from the donor to the recipient. In the early days of transplant surgery, this was viewed as a moral dilemma. Currently, if one accepts the definition of brain death, it is a medical dilemma.

This distinction between medical and moral dilemmas is also important in physicians' daily medical practices because most dilemmas occur in that setting. These dilemmas do not deal with terminal illnesses or severe injuries. They are less dramatic but far more common, because they arise from routine problems that everyone encounters to a greater or lesser extent. Even the treatment of a headache or stomachache can pose a dilemma if the physician does not elicit sufficient data to answer the patient's question. The type of treatment then decided on is based more on a value judgment than on what the data indicate the patient needs.

This is an easy habit to fall into, not only because these are common problems that physicians face, but also because physicians sometimes fear that they may open a Pandora's box of behavioral problems that must then be dealt with. Many physicians are uncomfortable in this area of patient care; some physicians take the position that dealing with behavioral problems is not even a function of physicians.

This is probably why the resolution of these kinds of dilemmas is often manifested in the prescribing habits of physicians. A prescription for medication substitutes for explaining to the patient the nature of the problem. Such a strategy may take several forms.

Termination behavior is one. The physician writes a prescription or orders an injection to conclude the visit with the patient and to move on to something else. It is irrelevant whether the medication is indicated for the condition. What is relevant is that the visit ends abruptly through the use of drugs. The patient may yet have unanswered questions, but the physician does not discover this because the visit has been concluded.

A second alternative is to prescribe something that the physician knows will have no direct effect on the patient's condition; the physician knows it to be an inert substance. In these instances, physicians usually imply that a diagnosis has been made and conclude by suggesting that the prescribed medication will either relieve the symptoms or cure the disease. This kind of treatment is called placebo therapy. The placebo effect is a very potent therapeutic force. The treatment is frequently successful, although sometimes the success is only short-lived.

Placebo therapy is usually criticized because the patient is being deceived. Not only is it demeaning to the patient to be deceived, but the deception also makes it impossible to obtain informed consent. A more important criticism may be, however, that the patient cannot be a participant in the treatment. For if the entire treatment is based on deception, how can the patient cooperate effectively in the cure?

A third method of prescribing medications is one that has attracted quite a bit of publicity in recent years. This is the use of nonspecific substances to treat symptoms that are caused by daily situations in life. Most commonly, the nonspecific substance prescribed is some form of psychoactive drug, usually a sedative or tranquilizer. The medication substitutes for a discussion of the problem, for an explanation of the development of the symptoms, and for suggestions that will help the patient learn to cope with the situation. This action is called mystification and has been described as follows:

> In the context of current usage drugs are medical agents whose function is the solution of medical problems. Only to the extent that interpersonal and other human problems can be construed as medical-psychiatric problems can they be considered appropriate targets for drug treatment. As more and more facets of human conduct, interactions, and conflict are considered to be "medical" problems physicians and, subsequently, patients become convinced that intervention through the medium of psychoactive drugs is desirable or required.[3]

We are creating a whole series of new problems by using psychoactive drugs in this rather vague and nonspecific manner. We are helping to create a belief that many life situations are illnesses amenable to treatment with drugs when the fact is that helping patients find ways of coping with the situations is more likely to be effective. In addition, the act of sedating the patient may reduce the patient's ability to cope effectively with adverse situations, thereby compounding the problem. Psychoactive drugs may sometimes be extremely useful aids in treating some patients, but they are not adequate substitutes for explaining to the patient the nature of the problem, nor are they substitutes for counseling the patient in how to cope with these situations.

[3] Henry L. Lennard, Leon J. Epstein, Arnold Bernstein, Donald C. Ransom, "Hazards Implicit in Prescribing Psychoactive Drugs," *Science*, July 31, 1970, vol. 169, pp. 438-441. Copyright 1970 by the American Association for the Advancement of Science.

The public must share somewhat in the responsibility for these kinds of dilemmas. In fact, the patient often creates the dilemma by implying or expressing the belief that counseling without an associated prescription would be ineffective. Nor is it uncommon for patients to go from one physician to another to obtain a prescription when they have been advised that other solutions would be more effective.

The poor resolution of these dilemmas may account for much of the criticism that is directed at the medical profession today. The functional incapacity of the patient is prolonged. Symptoms persist because the patient's questions are not answered satisfactorily. The use of resources increases as patients go elsewhere searching for answers to their problems. These dilemmas usually occur in patients with relatively ill-defined complaints—headaches, backaches, and so on. The common denominator is that all such symptoms require careful attention to the total patient rather than to a specific organ system if they are to be satisfactorily resolved.

The examples of prescribing habits certainly have moral overtones, particularly in regard to placebo therapy. Careful attention to the primary data will, however, usually permit the physician to assign a risk/benefit ratio to each decision strictly on the basis of the medical data. Even in these ill-defined areas, most dilemmas that occur can be defined as medical dilemmas rather than moral dilemmas and can be dealt with effectively.

All of this is further evidence that the role of the conceptually oriented physician is important. Expertise in acquiring primary data from the patient, in interpreting and evaluating them, and in synthesizing them with secondary data puts the primary physician in the best possible position to make decisions, understand the patient's priorities, and answer the patient's questions. Having acquired the data about the total patient and the patient's life situation, the primary physician is in a position to play a most important role in resolving the major dilemmas surrounding the use of medical technology, including drug therapy.

Multiphasic Screening 11

I remember seeing an elaborate and complicated automatic washing machine for automobiles that did a beautiful job of washing them. But it could do only *that, and everything else that got into its clutches was treated as if it were an automobile to be washed.*

Abraham H. Maslow, *The Psychology of Science*

This is an age of technology that we live in, and people have come to rely more and more on products and gadgets to do things that were once done in other ways. Engineering students used to use slide rules, but now they use calculators. And computers are almost within the reach of the middle class, computers that can do anything from controlling the temperature in homes to balancing checkbooks. Electric can openers are common. Television sets adjust their own color. Ovens clean themselves.

This superfluousness has also had some far-reaching effects in medicine. Recently, many health planners have begun to advocate increasing the use of technology as a physician substitute in order to reduce costs. Seymour Harris, for example, says, "A potentially significant approach to the shortage of physicians is to find lower cost substitutes such as the greater use of technology, capital, drugs, assistant physicians and technical personnel (including more highly trained nurses)."[1]

[1] Seymour E. Harris, *The Economics of Health Care—Finance & Delivery*, McCutchan Publishing Corp., Berkeley, Calif., 1975, p. 8.

Multiphasic screening has been proposed as one of these methods. Screening for disease is not a new concept in medical practice; it has been done by physicians to a greater or lesser extent for many decades. Whenever a physician performs a test on a patient that is unrelated to any of that patient's symptoms or physical findings, the physician is, in a sense, screening for a certain disease. Routine determination of the hemoglobin concentration, for example, as part of a general physical examination is a screen for the presence of anemia. Routine use of a tuberculin test is a screen for evidence of tuberculous infection. Routine performance of a Pap smear is a screen for cervical cancer. There are many other examples of screening in medical practice that have been employed for many years. Some of them are useful, some of them are controversial, and some of them have been shown to be useless. An example of a useless form of screening that was formerly widely used is routine X-ray examination of the upper and lower intestinal tract as a screen for intestinal cancer. It was gradually shown that the aggregate cost of this kind of examination and the relatively high radiation exposure were not justified by the low yield of cancer found. This examination is now performed only when symptoms suggest the possibility of disease, except in certain high-risk groups.

In general, screening could be viewed as a shortcut to diagnosis in patients without symptoms. Most often, a screen is set up in such a way that a single test is used either to exclude a certain disease or to initiate further studies in a patient who has a positive test. Some screens are highly successful and some are miserable failures. In all screens, however, the screener is working with limited amounts of data about the patients being tested. If this were not true, the tests would not be called screens.

Only in recent years has screening been looked at seriously as a physician substitute. It is advocated by many health planners and by some physicians, the primary justification being lower cost. While it is true that extensive screens have been devised whereby large numbers of patients can be tested for a variety of diseases at a very nominal cost, it has yet to be shown that the total cost (which includes the follow-up on the positive tests of the screen) would be lower. In fact, it is possible that the total cost of such a screen would be higher.

In the preceding chapters it was shown that physicians must work with large amounts of data in order to make decisions. Screening for disease does not provide such data. Most screens provide only one piece of information about any disease being tested for, and this is usually the result of a laboratory test. The large behavioral input by the patient during a medical interview is lost to the screener.

It is impossible to deal with patients effectively without extensive behavioral data, including the patients' concerns about diseases they may have, diseases they think they may have, interpersonal relationships, family relationships, and many other things. Patient care is ineffective without such data because patients' symptoms are often due to their concerns rather than their diseases. This is true even in major types of illnesses.

As an example, I once saw a young woman in consultation who had leg pains that had troubled her for many years. The pain began shortly after she recovered from a blood clot in the vein of that leg. She had been reassured many times that the original clot was not responsible for the pain she was having. She had also been reassured that she did not have a new clot to account for the pain. However, she did not experience any relief from her pain until she revealed in her medical history that she had an extreme fear of dying and that she had lived in fear of a sudden, fatal blood clot in her lungs since the original episode. Once this behavioral datum was determined, her fear could be dealt with and her symptoms disappeared.

Such data collecting is more time consuming than screening. But since most symptoms are associated with emotions as often as (or more often than) with diseases, it is less costly in the long run to deal with the emotions in conjunction with whatever diseases may be present.

Since multiphasic screening is being proposed as a substitute for physicians, it is important that the public understand how it is used and what its limitations are. Multiphasic screening is a form of testing designed to provide a large number of tests to a large number of people at a nominal cost. A large part of multiphasic screening consists of automated laboratory tests, but not all of the tests need be laboratory tests. For example, a multiphasic screen may consist of twelve to twenty automated laboratory tests that can be done inexpensively. In many situations, however, additional tests are added to this screen, such as blood pressure tests, breathing capacity tests, height and weight measurements, electrocardiograms (either resting or with exercise or both), chest X-rays, breast examinations in women, and so on. The specific tests in the screen are determined by the goals of the screening program and by the age and sex of the population being tested.

The proposal being made is that multiphasic screening be used in patient care as a form of triage to separate the patient population into various categories such as "well," "worried well," "early sick," and "sick."[2,3] Triage is a method used in massive disasters that aids physicians and nurses by rapidly classifying patients according to the extent of their wounds. Those who cannot be helped are

[2] Sidney H. Garfield, "The Delivery of Medical Care," *Scientific American*, April 1970, vol. 222, pp. 15–23.

[3] Morris F. Coleen, "Multiphasic Screening as a Triage to Medical Care," In *Controversy in Internal Medicine*, F. J. Ingelfinger et al., eds., vol. 2, W. B. Saunders Co., Philadelphia, 1974.

ignored, those who can be helped and need immediate attention get it, and those whose injuries can wait have to wait for medical attention. The use of the term triage by health planners, in fact, suggests the scope of the problem American medicine is facing, since this is a device that has hitherto been used only in massive natural disasters and wars.

While the use of multiphasic screening as a type of triage in patient care is superficially appealing, there are certain pitfalls associated with it. It is important that the public understand some of the limitations of screening if it is to be asked to decide whether to accept a screening mechanism as a substitute for the physician of first contact. To understand the concept of multiphasic screening, a distinction should be made between screening, case finding, and diagnostic examination. There are two reasons for making such a distinction. The first is that certain contractual considerations come into focus when mass screening is proposed. The second is that the predictive value (clinical reliability) of any particular laboratory test will vary considerably depending on whether the test is being used in a screening program or in a diagnostic evaluation.

The first major factor that distinguishes a screening program from case finding and from diagnostic evaluation is the nature of the patient population being studied. In screening programs, members of the public are actively solicited, by whomever is sponsoring the program, to be tested for a disease or a variety of diseases. In case finding and diagnostic evaluation the reverse is true: patients are soliciting advice from the physician concerning questions that they think the physician can answer.

This means that in mass screening the contract between the member of the public and the health facility is actually initiated by the health facility. This places a responsibility on the facility, and the nature of that responsibility must be understood by the public and by the sponsors of screening programs.

Implicit in the contract entered into by the sponsors of screening programs is that they are offering a test for a disease or for certain diseases that will enable them to tell the people being tested whether they probably have the disease. Also implicit in the contract is the understanding that diagnosis of the disease will make a difference to the person tested. If there is no effective treatment, no service has been performed by finding the condition. If the treatment is so drastic or so tedious that most patients without symptoms are not likely to comply with it, very little service has been performed. If the treatment is so complex or so unpleasant that patients in whom early diagnosis is made are likely to reject it, the test has not made any difference. If the disease being tested for is of a type that does not cause significant disability to the population being tested, the testing has not made any difference. It is also implicit in the contract made by the sponsors of screening programs that there are facilities in the community to confirm the positive tests and provide treatment.

Thus, one distinguishing characteristic of screening is that the contract is initiated by the sponsors of the program rather than by the people being tested. Another is that the people being tested are ostensibly healthy volunteers representing the general population.

Diagnostic evaluation of a patient falls at the other end of the spectrum. Diagnostic evaluations are initiated by the patients, and they are soliciting help from a physician to evaluate whatever is troubling them. They are not healthy volunteers from the general population, but individuals who seek medical advice to define the causes of their symptoms and to receive appropriate treatment. The physician's responsibility is to initiate a diagnostic study and to use whatever kinds of testing the physician deems appropriate to help define the problem. The use of tests is much more selective, and the justification for using the various tests is based on a different kind of contract made with the patient, namely, to find out what is wrong and then to recommend a treatment program if one is available.

Case finding falls somewhere between screening and diagnostic evaluation. A typical example of case finding is the individual who seeks medical counsel by requesting a periodic history and physical examination. Such patients may be free of symptoms or may have symptoms at the time of the examination. However, they come to the physician seeking clarification of their general status. In this situation, the physician usually employs certain laboratory tests as a routine part of a health evaluation regardless of the presence of symptoms. For example, the physician may employ certain tests designed to determine whether a cancer of the large bowel is present, even though the patient has no symptoms suggesting bowel disease. In a sense, some of the testing performed in case finding is not very different from the testing performed in mass screening except that the contract is initiated by the patient rather than the screener. The other difference between screening and case finding is that the patient who seeks medical counsel for periodic health evaluation is not necessarily a healthy volunteer representing the general population.

It is apparent that the contractual ramifications of screening are different from those of case finding or diagnostic evaluation. The kind of contract between the screening sponsor and the person being screened is different from that between the physician and the patient.

Another major difference between screening and case finding or diagnostic evaluation is that the predictive values of the tests vary considerably in each setting. This is particularly true if one compares screening to diagnostic evaluation.

Predictive value is the most important variable in

clinical medicine. As noted in Chapter 8, the predictive value is defined as the percentage of people with a positive test who actually have the disease. It defines the reliability of the test in the patient care setting. The predictive value of a test will be much higher when it is used to test a population for a disease with a high prevalence (a disease that is relatively common in the population group being studied) than when it is used to test a population with a low prevalence of the same disease. In the example in Chapter 8, the predictive value increased from 16 to 95 percent when the prevalence rose from 1 to 50 percent.

Clinicians exercise major control over the prevalence of the disease in the population they are testing. They are able to do this through the acquisition, interpretation, and synthesis of primary data as they perform histories and physical examinations on their patients. As skillful physicians acquire primary data sequentially from their patients (history, physical examination, preliminary testing) and as they synthesize these data with their secondary data (body of knowledge of medical practice), they are progressively narrowing the diagnostic possibilities and are increasing the likelihood that the disease for which they are going to test is the disease that the patient has. *In effect, they are moving the patient to be tested out of a population where the disease under consideration has a low prevalence into a population subgroup where the disease has a high prevalence. They are therefore increasing the predictive value of each test they use.* I daresay that with most common diseases, competent diagnosticians can, by performing careful histories and physical examinations, select people from the population consulting them in such a way that those selected have at least a 50 to 60 percent probability of having the disease under consideration before any specific laboratory testing is used. This means that the prevalence of the disease in the population being tested during a diagnostic evaluation is likely to be in the range of

50 to 60 percent, which is tremendously higher than the prevalence of that same disease being tested for in a screening program.

The importance of this concept cannot be overstated. The higher the frequency of occurrence of false positive tests, the higher the frequency of further needless repetitious testing with all of its attendant risk and expense. Anything that can reduce the number of erroneous laboratory results is bound to be in the public interest. Raising the predictive value of laboratory tests is one of the most effective ways of doing this.

It is important that the public know these differences between screening, case finding, and diagnostic evaluation. The major deficiency of screening in a patient care setting is that it is performed on subsets of the population without preliminary medical evaluation. Therefore, the prevalence of the disease being tested for in that population will be lower than the prevalence of the same disease in a subset selected from a population by the process of a diagnostic evaluation.

This is not to say that there is no place for screening in the health care system. On the contrary, mass screening can have considerable value, provided that it is used selectively and that the contractual implications of screening are noted and adhered to.

It is to say, however, that there are serious limitations to the use of multiphasic screening as a physician substitute and as a form of triage to separate the patient population into a variety of categories. The position that this kind of use of technology would reduce the cost of medical care must be carefully questioned. It is at least equally probable that using technology in this manner would result in a reduction of the quality of care and an increase of the total cost. Even when physicians are involved in the process of screening (physicians are involved in the triage recommendations cited above) they are involved only secondarily and are not the persons of first contact. Consequently, their data are quite different from the data they would acquire if they took the medical history personally. Since the medical history should provide some 75 percent of the useful primary data necessary to arrive at a diagnosis, and since 70 percent of the data acquired in this manner are thought to be nonverbal, it can be seen that much information is lost to physicians who acquire their information secondhand. In the absence of complete primary data, physicians become more reliant on testing. When this happens, the prevalence of a particular disease in the population under consideration becomes lower in direct proportion to the lack of primary data. As the prevalence goes down, the proportion of false positive tests goes up. In this manner, technology begets technology, and in situations involving patient care overuse of technology has many adverse implications.

What Is a Physician? 12

I will follow that method of treatment which, according to my ability and judgment, I consider for the benefit of my patients, and abstain from whatever is deleterious and mischievous.

Oath of Hippocrates

What is a physician? It is truly appalling to review the voluminous literature of proposed solutions to current problems in medical care and realize that they have all been developed without a definition of the role and function of the modern physician. Since it is generally agreed that the physician is the central figure in the health care apparatus, it seems elementary that the initial step toward resolving the current problems should be an attempt to provide such a definition. This would provide a solid base from which rational decisions about the use of various other health professionals as well as the use of certain kinds of modern technology could be made.

One reason why the question "What is a physician?" has not been examined in a critical and specific manner is probably that everyone thinks the answer is self-evident. Most of society (including physicians) continues to live with the pre-World War II image of the physician. This image was that any physician could fulfill the social mandate of the medical profession, which is that the physician be concerned with the maintenance and restoration of health. This popular image of the physician was probably never accurate, but it was a close enough representation. It fulfilled the public need in pre-World War II days because of the relative simplicity of the health care system.

The situation changed rapidly after World War II. Because of the increase in the capacity of medical technology, the health care apparatus became much more complex. Specialties proliferated. General practitioners attempted to use parts of the knowledge of technology of most of the specialties. Although the medical profession and the public were aware of these changes as they occurred, the long-term significance of the changes did not make the impact it should have. One of the results of this rapid change was that the modern physician could no longer be defined by the earlier broad generalization. Different physicians, because of their educational background and experience, had different functions and were working in entirely different ways.

In retrospect, this rapid proliferation of physicians with different kinds of functions had a chaotic effect on the medical profession and the public. As each new specialty developed, it defined the function of its members within the strictures of the body of knowledge of that specialty. As ever larger proportions of medical students chose to develop careers in these specialties and as the general practitioners became involved in multiple technologies, fewer physicians remained to fulfill the broad public mandate of the physician's function to maintain and restore health. This caused internal strife in the medical profession. Some physicians felt that specialists could continue to perform the broad function of the physician as well as the specialist function. Other physicians thought the specialists were unable to perform this dual function. It also caused some strife between the medical profession and the public as the public became aware that not all of their expectations of physicians were being fulfilled.

The function of the modern physician has become so complex that it will never again be possible to define the physician's function in a way that will apply to all physicians. Medical practice has, of necessity, become increasingly fragmented with the proliferation of the specialties. The specialties, in turn, have proliferated because of the impressive increase in medical technology since the end of World War II. This leaves two alternative ways of answering the question "What is a physician?"

The first alternative is to formalize the movement that has been occurring spontaneously since the end of World War II, namely to define the physician's function within the confines of each separate, newly developed specialty. A neurosurgeon would then be defined by the ability to perform within the limits of that specialty, as would a dermatologist, ophthalmologist, radiologist, and so forth. This is a useful and accurate method of defining a physician's function. As a matter of fact, it is the method that is used within the profession to help physicians decide on whom to call for a consultation. However, this definition is not very useful to the public. Its shortcoming becomes apparent when one considers that there are eleven recognized specialty areas within the field of internal medicine alone.

It would be a formidable task for a patient to have to deal with such a large number of definitions when seeking help for a specific complaint. Suppose, for example, a patient has a stomach pain. That pain could be treated by a number of specialists, such as the primary physician, the general surgeon, the gastroenterologist, the vascular surgeon, the gynecologist, the urologist, the endocrinologist, the cardiologist, the immunologist, the psychiatrist, the hematologist, or the colon-rectal surgeon. Equally imposing lists could be made for other common symptoms, such as chest pain, back pain, headache, and so on. For this reason, defining a physician's function according to specialty is not useful for the public, even though it is useful for the medical profession.

The second alternative is to look at the broad function of physicians as that function relates to the public need. Earlier in this book I noted that the historic generalist-specialist distinction has become useless as a means of providing a definition of the physician's function because nearly all graduating physicians are now specialists. It has also become detrimental by adding more to confusion than to clarity in the public mind. The observation was made that modern physicians can be divided into two broad categories, the conceptually oriented and the technologically oriented physicians. All of the specialties fall into one of these two broad classifications.

In general, the technologically oriented physician belongs to groups of physicians who have limited their expertise to either a single organ system or the application of a certain type of technology (surgery, radiology, pathology, gastroenterology, dermatology, hematology, and so on). The technologically oriented physicians' function within the medical profession is very well defined. Their public image is also well defined. These physicians perform an important and useful function in patient care, mostly in the diagnosis and treatment of certain uncommon diseases or uncommon manifestations of common diseases, and sometimes in the care of patients who are extremely ill with diseases that fall within their specialty. They also perform a useful and important function by providing certain kinds of instrumentation that are used in the diagnostic or therapeutic process and by providing expertise in the use of some complex and dangerous forms of nonsurgical treatment. With technologically oriented physicians, then, the question "What is a physician?" is not a problem. The function of physicians of this kind is well defined and their importance and usefulness in the overall schema are well established.

The name of the game in medical practice is, however, patient care. This means care of the total patient as well as treatment of any disease the patient may have. The technologically oriented physician is usually neither a physician of first contact nor one in a position to provide continuing care and to assume continuing responsibility for the total patient. Therefore, defining the role and function of the technologically oriented physician is not sufficient to completely answer the question of what a physician is.

The members of the various commissions that issued reports in the early and middle 1960s about this problem (Coggeshall report, Millis report, Willard report, National Advisory Commission of Health Manpower report) exhibited considerable wisdom and vision. Of these, the writers of the Millis report seem to have made a more explicit effort to define the role and function of the physician. It was in the Millis report that the term "primary physician" originated. Of the existing specialties, general internal medicine, general pediatrics, and family medicine come closest to the definition of the primary physician. Most of the descriptive data, provided in the earlier chapters of this book, about the activities of the physician in a daily practice relate to the activities of the primary physician. In other words, conceptually oriented physicians and what has come to be called primary physicians are synonymous.

What, then, are conceptually oriented (primary) physicians?

They are managers. If medicine is a conceptual science that uses technology when indicated, the implication is strong that there has to be someone who decides in each instance when the various forms of technology are indicated and when they are not. This is one of the functions of primary physicians if they are properly educated for the task.

They gather, interpret, and evaluate data and synthesize primary data with secondary data. The main tools used by primary physicians are various forms of data (both primary data acquired from the patient and secondary data—their fund of general knowledge). Their primary data do not exclude any organ system of the body and concern the total person in that person's social environment. In order to use these tools effectively, they also have to be experts in interpreting data, evaluating them, and synthesizing these two kinds of data. The acquisition and use of these data are not simple. This is particularly true in the acquisition of primary data, of which the medical history plays a major part. In order to obtain an accurate medical history, the physician must be able to relate well to the patient, attend carefully to the total demeanor of the patient as well as to the verbal history, and interpret accurately the meaning of what the patient is saying. There are also many sources of error in the interpretation of laboratory findings as well as in the logic of making decisions, and the physician must be aware of these. All of these skills must be superimposed on an extensive knowledge of disease manifestations and of human behavior.

They are decision makers. Throughout the physician-patient interaction, the primary physician is making decisions. These include decisions about when enough studies have been performed and when and what kind of treatment is necessary.

They are probability experts. In patient care there is no fixed recipe that can be followed in treating a particular disease. Patient care consists of sequential decision making. The decisions must then be implemented in the face of the uncertainty caused by continuing change in the patient and also by the fact that patients with the same type of illness vary considerably. In order to make the sequential decisions, physicians must be probability experts. In a sense, they are odds makers for their patients—highly skilled and educated ones, to be sure, but odds makers nonetheless. They base their estimates of the outcome on an extensive body of knowledge plus their previous experiences with similar types of problems. Since outcome is nearly always uncertain, their decisions are usually directed toward providing the most optimal risk/benefit ratio for their patients.

They are therapists. At the conclusion of the diagnostic process, the primary physician must make a decision about treatment. Multiple options are open. The first decision concerns whether the physician should treat the patient or refer the patient to a technologically oriented physician. If the physician decides to treat the patient, the second decision concerns whether the best treatment consists of counseling the patient, prescribing medication, or both.

These roles, then, define the primary physician as a physician who can meet public expectations as well as one who can fill the social role consistently and effectively. A difficult task? Of course. And it is rendered more difficult because the target of the physician's decisions is a fellow human being. Otto Guttentag wrote:

> In medicine object and subject, i.e., patient and physician, are fellow human beings. They are equals in the ontological sense. In other professions of care, e.g., maintenance engineering, veterinary medicine or pastoral care, objects and subjects differ. Machines are completely cognitively transparent, men are not; animals are inferior to man in terms of human rationality; God or whatever name we may give to the object of our unconditional loyalty is superior. Speaking in terms of practicality, physicians do not know more about patients than they know about themselves.[1]

All the foregoing seems imposing, but it is not unattainable. To be sure, the primary physician must be a highly educated person. However, by augmenting the required knowledge base with greater emphasis on the

[1] Otto E. Guttentag, "Medical Humanism: A Redundant Phrase," *Pharos*, January 1969, vol. 32, pp. 12–15. Reprinted with the permission of the editor.

broad aspects of medicine and by eliminating the necessity to learn to perform various kinds of medical technology (because the technological skills can be provided by technologically oriented physicians), the conceptually oriented physician can be educated to a high degree of knowledge and skill in the same length of time as the technologically oriented physician. A diagram helps clarify some of these activities (see Fig. 1).

Acceptance of this definition of the function of the primary physician would benefit society in several ways. First, an unexpected bonus would be that the technologically oriented physician would be made more effective by such a change. Highly skilled primary physicians would concentrate prevalence to a high degree, higher by far than is achieved through patient self-referral to a technologically oriented physician and higher than is possible with the various forms of triage. Consider, for example, the group of patients referred to an endocrinologist by such physicians to confirm the diagnosis of metabolic disease. This group would have a much lower proportion of false positive tests, and the necessity for further testing would be reduced.

For too long the public has sustained the illusion that patient care is an exact science. By and large it is not. The perpetuation of this illusion has been a disservice to the public and to the medical profession because it frequently causes unrealistic expectations of outcome on the part of the patient and the physician. Unfortunately, when these expectations are present, they not only lead to disappointment of the patient, the physician, and the patient's family, but also increase the cost of medical care by encouraging needless overuse of services.

Second, if the primary physician becomes the physician of first contact for all patients, and continues to assume responsibility for the same patients, health care costs will be reduced. They will be reduced because there will be more realistic decision making in which the probabilities of

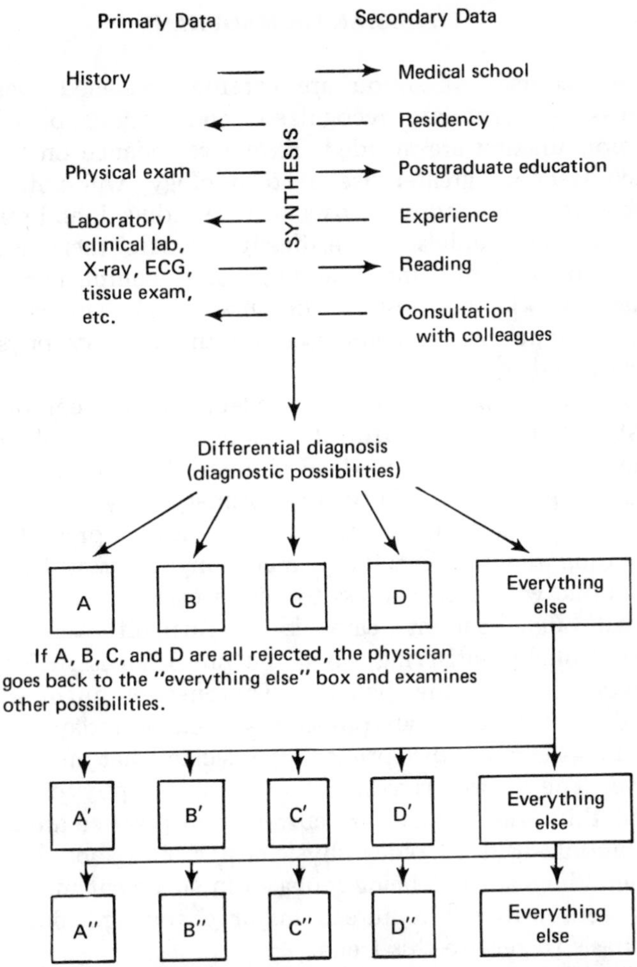

Figure 1 The diagnostic process. Each increment of differential diagnostic possibilities is associated with less common diseases and/or increasingly difficult problems. At some point (depending on the experience and educational background of the physician), consultation is requested. The process is really more complex than indicated here. At each stage of the differential diagnostic progression, the physician goes back to the top of the diagram and obtains additional history, reexamines the patient, and reviews the need for additional laboratory studies.

various courses of action are carefully weighed, possible sources of error are recognized, and various pitfalls of decision making are avoided. Extensive reliance on testing, which leads to greater use of technology, will not occur. Both direct and indirect costs will be reduced, and services will not be duplicated needlessly because there will be increased patient understanding and compliance. This reduction will be possible because of the much larger primary data base accumulated by the primary physician initially and over time.

Finally, it will provide an intellectually and emotionally satisfying form of medical practice, which will cause increasing numbers of medical students to want to become primary physicians. Since the primary physician is the medical specialist in shortest supply at the present time, increasing the numbers of primary physicians will provide the public with easier access to health care.

Although patient care is a difficult task, it is proportionally satisfying when the physician is sufficiently prepared to meet the challenge. The question might well be asked whether there are physicians available today to fulfill the functions of the primary physician that are defined above. The answer is yes, but most of the physicians who fulfill this function and are currently in practice are among the middle-aged to older physicians. For reasons discussed earlier, they are not being replaced in sufficient numbers as they retire. It will require a major change in educational emphasis to reverse this trend.[2]

We have discussed a workable definition of conceptually oriented physicians in terms of function. For the definition to be complete, however, it must also include the role of these physicians in the health care system—how they are

[2] Daniel F. Whiteside, "Training the Nation's Health Manpower—The Next Four Years," *Public Health Reports*, March–April 1977, vol. 92, pp. 99–107.

viewed by the public and their colleagues. It is clear in the definition of function that these are the physicians of first contact for the patient, that they are responsible for most of the major decisions affecting the welfare of their patients, and that they accept this responsibility indefinitely. Implicit in the definition is the fact that they should be given the commensurate authority to enable them to fulfill their responsibility. It is not enough, however, that the authority be implicit. It must be made explicit if the public desires to have physicians willing to undertake these responsibilities. The analogy has been made that the primary physician has the same role in medical practice that the captain has on board ship or that a chief executive officer of a corporation has within the corporate structure. That analogy breaks down, however, because the lines of authority are not as clearly defined in medical practice as they are in the other two situations.

It is to reverse this trend that redefining the physician's role and function is being suggested. It is imperative that authority commensurate with responsibility be returned to primary physicians by the profession as well as by society to enable them to fulfill their role as the overall managers of the care of their patients. Otherwise, not only will the relatively small number of primary physicians be fairly ineffective, but it will not be a specialty attractive to medical students.

Conclusion 13

What is totally new, however, and in contradiction to all the modern university has ever believed, is the shift away from the disciplines as the center of teaching and learning. But this was bound to happen as application became central to knowledge.

Peter F. Drucker, *The Age of Discontinuity*

Virtually everybody has heroes, and I am no exception. The heroes one chooses are normally quite influential in determining the positions one takes throughout life and what one will become. Two of my heroes are from the medical past, and they have had a great influence on the thoughts I have presented in this book. They are little known outside the medical profession, and one is little known inside the medical profession. They are Thomas Sydenham and Pierre Louis.

Thomas Sydenham was the better known of the two. This seventeenth century Englishman was a keen observer and had an extremely analytical mind. Known as the English Hippocrates, he formalized the recording and study of the natural history of diseases. He recognized that physicians could not evaluate the effectiveness of treatment until they first recorded the behavior of a disease without treatment; only then could anyone say whether treatment made a difference. As a result of his observations, he became increasingly critical of many of the forms of treatment that were used during his lifetime. At one point he wrote, and this statement has great relevance even today, that in many instances, "I have consulted my own patients safely and my own reputation most effectively by doing nothing at all."[1]

Pierre Louis was a nineteenth century Frenchman and is considered to be the father of modern biostatistics. In a way, he extended and refined Sydenham's methods. His work led to the rejection of the then popular forms of treatment consisting of bloodletting and the application of leeches for many diseases. At the time, that was quite an advance.

Modern medical knowledge in the areas in which these two were pioneers makes their advances and concepts seem almost primitive today. They did, however, lay the foundation for later advances. In most major advances, while the initial breakthroughs may have been technological, the ultimate breakthroughs have been conceptual. The conceptual breakthroughs have provided the path by which the technological advances may be used to their greatest advantage. Today we need another conceptual breakthrough, since the potential for both harm and good from modern medical, diagnostic, and therapeutic technology is so great that physicians need access to the most sophisticated methods of evaluation in order to achieve optimal patient care.

The question that people should be asking today about health care in this country is "To what extent is medical technology being overused?" There is no easy way to answer that question, but there are some figures available that suggest that the use of medical technology has grown enormously. In 1929 $3.6 billion was spent on health care, and in 1976 this figure jumped to $139.3 billion. In 1929

[1] Ralph H. Major, *Classic Descriptions of Disease*, Charles C Thomas, Springfield, Ill., 1945, p. 195.

18.1 percent of this amount was spent on hospital services and 27.7 percent on physicians' services. In 1974 the corresponding percentages were 39.2 and 18.2. Looked at another way, the proportion of the national health expenditure used for hospital services increased 63 times over a 45-year period, while the proportion used for physicians' services increased 19 times in the same period.

The nature of hospital care changed significantly during these years. Before World War II, hospital care for either the acutely ill or the chronically ill was often a domiciliary type of care, somewhat comparable to that in nursing homes today. Currently, hospital care is received largely by patients needing a variety of sophisticated forms of medical technology. So one interpretation of these figures is that they simply reflect the increased use of medical technology that has been developing since World War II.

These figures represent only the direct cost of health services—the cost for services rendered, ranging from services for health care to the construction of health care facilities to the cost of research. A less well-known figure is the indirect cost of the health care system, the cost of lost productivity due to disability or early death. The indirect cost is usually estimated to be about twice the direct cost.

But estimates of indirect cost are based only on death or disability from illnesses that have an organic cause. I have never been able to find any estimates of the total cost that include the cost of disabilities of psychosomatic origin. Their inclusion could increase these estimates almost exponentially since about two-thirds of the problems physicians see are emotional in origin.

The fact remains that direct cost alone is the major stimulus responsible for present efforts to change the structure of the health care system. That is probably why most of the proposed solutions emphasize mainly the reduction of direct cost, and all proposals focus on lowering unit costs while allowing demand to increase. The results of this narrow focus can be far-reaching, for if direct cost were reduced in such a way that indirect cost rose, the reduction in direct cost would represent a Pyrrhic victory for society. The resulting total cost would be larger than ever. Containing the direct cost by appropriately reducing the use of diagnostic and therapeutic technology would be desirable, and this is where we should be looking.

So far, most of the suggestions for changing the structure of the health care system have been directed toward changing the point of entry into the system. Traditionally, the physician has served this function, and the process of entering the system has been associated with the performance of a history and physical examination. Various proposals, however, suggest that cost could be reduced by replacing the physician as the point of entry with a less well-trained substitute. These alternatives are based on the principle of triage—sorting patients into various categories and then either dismissing them or treating them.

Technology would play a major role in these proposals. Usually, the patient's history would be obtained by an automated or semiautomated method, followed by several tests and measurements. All of these studies would be performed by technical personnel. Then, on completion of the study, a physician would review the data and make a decision about the patient's health. In one proposal, the patient would be judged to be well, worried well, early sick, or sick. Many of these tests, however, would not be applicable to each individual patient. Their accuracy would be suspect because the predictive values of the tests would be low.

The original stimulus for using physician assistants as the health professionals of first contact for patients in triage probably originated in the military services during World War II. Medical corpsmen were widely used for this purpose, and because it was reasonably successful in the military setting, it was proposed as a solution in the civilian setting. But it should be pointed out that there is quite a difference between the military and the civilian population. Military personnel, especially in time of war, are mostly young and healthy and are examined quite thoroughly before their induction. Many diseases will not be found in this population to any large degree, and so the chance of a medical corpsman committing a grievous error is not very large.

In the civilian setting, however, the risk of misinterpreting important data from the history or physical examination is much greater. The evaluation of a patient with chest pain is one example where the subtleties of history taking can be of vital importance to the patient. A chest pain may be completely innocuous, or it may be indicative of a critical emergency where the patient may die in moments. A patient who comes to a clinic with symptoms of fatigue and who is found to be anemic is another example of the importance of careful interpretation and evaluation of the primary data. Anemia may be a simple problem, easily resolved, or it may be caused by serious internal bleeding, by a variety of forms of cancer, by certain kinds of primary blood diseases, or by various other diseases. If such a patient were to be given iron treatment on the assumption that the anemia was of a simple kind, valuable time might be lost that could make the difference in whether the patient's problem was treatable or untreatable.

When triage is used as a substitute for a careful examination by a physician, there is also the risk that the true concerns of the patient will not be discovered. This is particularly true if the method does not disclose an organic problem to explain the symptoms. When this happens, patients usually seek advice from other physicians or health professionals. A person with a chronic headache, for example, can be dealt with in one of two ways. One is by a physician taking a careful and detailed history of the headache problem, obtaining the social, behavioral, and past medical history that is related to the problem. The physician will also take a general medical history and then perform a careful physical examination. Acquiring this data takes about an hour; only then will the physician begin to think of the necessity of obtaining more primary data by using laboratory studies or by consulting other specialists.

This physician knows that 95 percent of headache problems are associated with emotional stress and is therefore in a position to deal with the majority of headache problems. But the physician also knows, since the appropriate data have been acquired, when the patient's problem is not caused by emotions.

The second common way to deal with a patient who has chronic headaches is for a health professional of first contact to refer the patient to another professional, usually a technologically oriented physician. When this happens, the referral is usually made because of inadequate experience of the professional of first contact or because of inadequate acquisition of primary data. Sometimes, too, the patient consults a technologically oriented physician first.

Once the patient is committed to this method, a common sequence is for the patient to be referred first to an ophthalmologist and then to a neurologist; frequently, a variety of laboratory studies are performed, such as brain scans and electroencephalograms, and sometimes even invasive procedures such as lumbar punctures and cerebral angiography are used. While all these studies are appropriate for certain kinds of headache problems, they are not appropriate as screening devices. They are time-consuming, sometimes invasive and dangerous, and always expensive.

At a certain point, the symptoms can become fixed in some patients. This means that the patient begins to think there must be something seriously wrong to warrant all the studies and consultations that have taken place. It becomes much more difficult to counsel such a patient should the headache later prove to be caused by emotional problems. Once the symptoms become fixed, the patient becomes an inveterate doctor-user and adds considerably to the total demand for medical care. Direct and indirect costs rise.

The assumption behind the use of triage in the health care system is that the demands on the system will grow indefinitely. And indeed they will if a patient's particular problems, especially the emotionally induced ones, are not dealt with effectively when that patient first sees a physician. But it is quite likely that if there were an adequate number of well-trained primary physicians, the demands on the health care system could be contained. Patients would not think it necessary to seek the services of several physicians to have their problems explained. This would, of course, require that physicians deal satisfactorily with all of their patient's problems.

In addition, if all patients' problems were dealt with more satisfactorily and more personally, it is possible that other criticisms of the medical profession, such as that physicians are inaccessible or impersonal and dehumanizing, would be diminished. Patients would not be shuffled from clinic to clinic or from doctor to doctor. One doctor would be able to treat most patients' problems, referring them to other physicians only when the data indicated that it was necessary. Possibly more physicians, if they were taught the dynamics of the patient-physician interaction, would be available to the public because they would find it a rewarding way to practice medicine.

The most far-reaching decisions are made during the initial contact between patients and the health care system. That is why triage is an inadequate response to the present problems in patient care. It is at this point that the patient is sent on an almost irretrievable course toward either rational treatment or a long chain of diagnostic and therapeutic excesses. A conceptually oriented physician is the one who can decide on a rational course of treatment; therefore, this physician should be the patient's first contact with the health care system.

I want to emphasize that this is not an antitechnology book, nor am I opposed to technology. I use technology in my medical practice daily and recognize its importance. Medical technology has greatly extended the capacity of the modern physician. But technology must be guided. To date, its use has been dictated largely by its existence. This I oppose. Its overuse has become an abuse, not just of the technology, but of the faith of the public in the medical profession. Conceptualists—physicians who can control these excesses—are needed. They must be broadly educated, and they must become a sort of patient advocate. They must monitor and control the use of technology.

There are two major points I want to make in this book. The first is that the crisis in patient care can be traced to the gradual and unrecognized division of the role and function of the American physician into two separate entities. Nearly all physicians today are specialists; so this is not the traditional generalist-specialist division. Instead, it is the separation of technological and conceptual functions. The technologists and their role are established solidly in society. Only recently, however, has the need for conceptually oriented physicians been recognized. It is now time to begin educating this type of physician in earnest.

The second point follows directly from the first. Conceptually oriented physicians, because of the unique training they would receive, should always be the health professionals of first contact. Other, more technological contacts should be used only as adjuncts in patient care. These conceptually oriented physicians should also be given the authority commensurate with their responsibilities for long-term, continuing care of patients. Physicians of this type would also help reduce the unrealistic expectations of outcome in patient care.

A great deal of lip service has been given to the idea of primary care during the past several years, but only a minimum of serious planning and implementation of educational programs has occurred. A major reason for this is probably the failure, thus far, to define the role and function of the primary physician. The absence of a well-defined role and function makes it difficult to define a teachable body of knowledge. The underlying problem is that physicians, even those in the primary care specialties, cannot seem to agree on what primary physicians should do, how they should be trained, or how they would fit into the educational establishment. As an example, consider the following quotations from the *Archives of Internal Medicine* in its report on a Conference on the Role and Training of the General Internist.

> Because of the very diversity of his interest, the general internist is placed in a position analogous to Buridan's ass that starved to death because it could make no choice when confronted by equally appealing sources of nourishment.[2]

> Certainly in the past ten or fifteen years, it took an unusually sanguine person to think that there was any hope for a career in general internal medicine in the salaried faculty ranks, and especially in the tenured ranks, of most departments of medicine.[3]

> Another view is that internal medicine has become so complex and so demanding that to ask of the physician-internist to assume this very exacting role is not congruent with medicine's

[2]Stephen E. Goldfinger, "Continuing Education and General Internal Medicine," *Archives of Internal Medicine*, September 9, 1977, vol. 137, p. 1314. Copyright 1977, American Medical Association.

[3]Daniel Federman, "The General Internist as a Faculty Member," *Archives of Internal Medicine*, September 9, 1977, vol. 137, p. 1323. Copyright 1977, American Medical Association.

> recent successes. Perhaps we should turn this role over to somebody else.... At least one potential outgrowth of such a course might be to train two kinds of physicians: those who practice simple front-line medicine and those who carry on the complex kinds of goals that are traditionally pursued by the internist.[4]

> Third, given our disagreements among ourselves in perception of what the product [the general internist] ought to be, writing a uniform entry or certifying examination instrument proves to be very difficult.[5]

After reading this book, the reader should be able to see how these quotations exemplify some of the problems in patient care. There is no well-defined body of knowledge for teaching its subtleties. General internists are expected to perform as technologists if they wish to succeed in an academic setting; the role model for students then becomes a technologically oriented rather than a conceptually oriented physician. There appears to be little future for the general internist in the academic setting. In fact, it is suggested that the general internist be limited to "simple front-line medicine" while subspecialists are to assume the "complex kinds of goals that are traditionally pursued by the internist."

The same problems exist in the other two primary care specialties, pediatrics and family medicine. Perhaps one should stop and ask why this confusion about the role of conceptually oriented physicians exists. It exists in large part because this kind of physician is no longer accepted as

[4] From a paper by David E. Rogers, given to a discussion group on "The Role and Training of the General Internist," *Archives of Internal Medicine*, September 9, 1977, vol. 137, p. 1331. Copyright 1977, American Medical Association.

[5] Daniel Federman, quoted in "The Role and Training of the General Internist," *Archives of Internal Medicine*, September 9, 1977, vol. 137, p. 1334. Copyright 1977, American Medical Association.

a worthy faculty member, for the reasons stated in Chapter 4. At present, this kind of physician has no future in medical education.

A different attitude is required if the educational system is to change in the foreseeable future. This may come only with difficulty, because we are talking about changing an educational paradigm in which large numbers of people have a heavy investment.

Such a change must be carefully planned. Educational programs for the conceptually oriented physician of the future must be given high priority. The educational content must assure that such physicians continue to be required to maintain at least the same high standards of basic knowledge of disease as do their current counterparts. In addition, teaching the behavioral and analytical tools described in this book should be incorporated into their curriculum. Present members of medical school faculties would have to accept as peers new faculty members with interests different from their own. These new faculty members would include primary physicians as well as nonphysicians who are experts in behavioral and analytical sciences. Such a change would indicate that American medicine is at last heading in the direction of providing a place for conceptually oriented physicians in the medical profession.

Medicine is not and never has been an exact science, but today many people, including physicians, think it is. Indeed, patient care would be much simpler if for every problem there were a demonstrable cause, and if for every cause there were a specific, effective treatment. That is not the case, however. The human body is simply too complex, and it would take a magician to make it otherwise. In the simplest terms, that is why there should be conceptually oriented physicians controlling the use of medical technology. They would be knowledgeable in the traditional, biomedical aspects of patient care as well as the conceptual aspects. To have access to such a physician today would probably be one of the greatest breakthroughs in patient care, particularly since most of the primary physicians in practice now are middle-aged or older and are not being replaced by adequate numbers of younger physicians. No drama would be involved, and establishing a solid educational program would not make headlines.

But, as the Millis report said, "It is time for a revolution in the education of the primary physician, not a few patchwork adaptations."

Index